Prognosis HOPE

Prognosis
HOPE

*A Care Givers and Care Seekers
Guide to Em1powered Care*

Angie Felts, RN

NEW YORK

LONDON • NASHVILLE • MELBOURNE • VANCOUVER

Prognosis HOPE
A Care Givers and Care Seekers Guide to Em1powered Care

Published in New York, New York, by Morgan James Publishing. Morgan James is a trademark of Morgan James, LLC. www.MorganJamesPublishing.com

ISBN 978-1-64279-348-2 paperback
ISBN 978-1-64279-349-9 eBook
Library of Congress Control Number: 2018913197

Cover Design by:
Rachel Lopez
www.r2cdesign.com

Interior Design by:
Bonnie Bushman
The Whole Caboodle Graphic Design

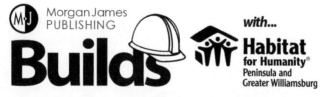

In an effort to support local communities, raise awareness and funds, Morgan James Publishing donates a percentage of all book sales for the life of each book to Habitat for Humanity Peninsula and Greater Williamsburg.

Get involved today! Visit
www.MorganJamesBuilds.com

"Each time a man stands up for an ideal, or acts to improve the lot of others, or strikes out against injustice, he sends forth a tiny ripple of hope, and crossing each other from a million different centers of energy and daring, those ripples build a current that can sweep down the mightiest walls of oppression and resistance."

—Robert Kennedy

Table of Contents

Foreword   *ix*

Acknowledgement   *xi*

Chapter 1   Divine Intervention   1

Chapter 2   But Wait, There's More!   9

Chapter 3   Puzzle Pieces   15

Chapter 4   Blended By Love   21

Chapter 5   I Surrender   27

Chapter 6   The Power of Human Connection   35

Chapter 7   Eating Their Young   41

Chapter 8   Opportunity Knocks   49

Chapter 9   Participation Required   53

Chapter 10   Empower to the People   59

Chapter 11   Identity Theft   65

Chapter 12   Disguised Blessing   69

Chapter 13   Second Chances   75
Chapter 14   People not Patients   81
Chapter 15   Alabama   87
Chapter 16   Losing Marbles   93
Chapter 17   3:22   99
Chapter 18   Fostering Hope   105
Chapter 19   Darkness Before Light   113
Chapter 20   Saving Pearl   121
Chapter 21   More Than Enough   129
Chapter 22   Mystery Diagnosis   135
Chapter 23   Closing the Gap   143
Chapter 24   Opportunity For All   151

In Memory of Shelley Moriston   161
About the Author   163

Foreword

As the president of the National Nurses in Business Association, I have the honor to see nurses creating needed services, products, and programs that impact and improve people's lives. In today's healthcare market place, much improvement is needed. What once were community hospitals have been closed or have been acquired into mega corporate systems. Technology and Big Data are increasing de-humanization and decreasing the time actually spent working and connecting with patients. The attrition of nursing graduates and burnout levels in the healthcare workforce is at all-time highs. *Both* the care-givers and the care-seekers are becoming increasingly vulnerable.

It is this vulnerable population that Angie's book so beautifully addresses, and she has developed a solution called the Prognosis HOPE Method. Through very personal stories of her life, colleagues, mentors, and patients, Angie shares what evolved as a positive action that results in empowerment of all the individuals involved.

Angie wants to reach care-givers and care-seekers with her message believing that *Prognosis HOPE* can restore meaningful connections and by doing so heal a fractured healthcare delivery system. By the end of Angie's book, you will want to stand up and cheer and be part of the prognosis hope revolution.

—Michelle DeLizio Podlesni RN

President National Nurses in Business Association ,

Author of *Unconventional Nurse® Going from Burnout to Bliss!*

Acknowledgement

When I think about **Human Connection**, the people that come to mind first are my parents, Linda and Bill. They brought me into this world under less than perfect circumstances and they both did the very best they could for my sister and me. My Mom read every word I wrote and gave me encouragement as each chapter unfolded. Although my Dad passed away before this book was complete, I know it would have made him proud. My sister, Korey, was my childhood partner in crime. We often found ourselves in deep water due to our curious nature. Now in our fifties, most of that mischief has been passed down to our sons, Anthony, Nick and Alec. No matter what, through our ups and downs, she was and will always be my first trusted friend.

Opportunity has come to me in many ways over my lifetime. Since I became a registered nurse, Gina, my business partner, has given me one of the biggest opportunities of my career. I have the honor of working with seniors in a way I always dreamed of. Even better, our partnership has grown into a friendship and has given me the opportunity to be a mentor to her daughters Cassy and Ally. There has been no greater opportunity though, than to be Anthony's mom and Todd's wife. These two loves of my life have forever changed me for the better. They have given me the opportunity to give and receive unconditional love. This gift has healed me in ways I could never imagine. Todd and Anthony will always represent what I hold most dear in my life.

I've always thought of myself as someone who participates. I'm not the kind of girl that sits on the sidelines. I'm all in, all the time. When it came to writing this book, my **Participation** was quite different. I started and stopped a lot over the last ten years. It really wasn't until I began sharing my writing with other people that I went all in. Please know that if you were one of those people, your feedback meant the world to me. One person in particular stands out. She is one of my biggest cheerleaders and also happens to be my editor, Katy Carpenter, owner of The Content Artist. Katy, thank you for not only believing in my message, but also making sure readers would hear my voice.

When it comes to **Empowerment**, there are people who have recently entered my life that have given me the confidence to move forward in ways that I had never imagined possible. Kane Minkus, President of Industry Rockstar, taught me to play bigger. His team of mentors has been amazing and I appreciate their guidance so much. Kane is also responsible for putting this next person on my radar. David Hancock, Founder and CEO of Morgan James Publishing believed in me when I was just starting to. His enthusiasm about *Prognosis HOPE* was the spark I needed to move forward with my dream of becoming an author. I am incredibly grateful to the entire team at Morgan James Publishing for their support in helping me get my message out to the world. Sometimes the best way to empower someone is to inspire that person. From the moment I met Michelle Podlesni, President of the National Nurses in Business Association, I was inspired. As a nurse, leader, entrepreneur, author and coach she empowers all nurses to find unconventional ways to be their very best. She is the beacon for us all on a horizon full of endless possibilities.

There is no doubt in my mind that when I needed **Hope** in my life my Grandpa was the one I turned to most often. When I was young, it was his gentle encouragement that everything would be all right. As I grew older, he was the foundation I could come back to when I felt lost. He was there for me during my darkest hours and because of him I had the courage to survive. Once again, when I was at the biggest crossroads of my life, he came through for me. He knew just the right words to share with me so I could finally begin my true-life path. One week before he passed unexpectedly, I gave him my word that I would become a nurse. That promise will always be one of the best ones I ever made.

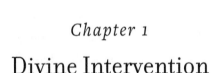

Chapter 1

Divine Intervention

*"You are full of unshaped dreams...you are
laden with beginnings...there is hope in you..."*
–Lola Ridge

A s I pulled over into the emergency lane, with steam coming up through the hood, I was so disappointed that once again my journey to college was being delayed. Only a week before, my car had overheated for the first time. The engine had gotten so hot that the block actually cracked, and the engine had to be rebuilt. If this had been any other car, I might have just left it behind. However, this was no ordinary car. She was the "Green Queen", a 1969 Cougar with a 351 Cleveland engine under her hood and I had worked three jobs to pay for her. This was the car that would be with me through college and medical school. At the ripe old age of 19, she was my prized possession. She was also a reminder to me that hard work paid off and when you wanted something you go after it and give it your all. The guy I bought her from only wanted $1,800.00. He gave me three months to come up with the money. When I handed him the cash, before the 90 days were up, he seemed pretty impressed. He gave me the keys and said, "This car is old, but solid, and if you take care of her, she will take care of you." I gave him my word that I would take really good care of her and told him about the journey ahead for me and the Green Queen.

That journey began with a cross-country road trip from California to Pennsylvania. I had been accepted into the University of Pittsburgh, where I would complete my Bachelor of Science degree and then hoped to head to medical school after that. Cindy, my best friend from middle school, had flown into San Diego to do the road trip with me. We thought we'd have a little fun before we both had to get serious about our college careers. My mom, Linda, had decided to relocate back to her home state of Pennsylvania, so she would also be making the trip with us. Our plan was to drop Cindy off in Missouri, where she currently lived, and my mom and I would continue to Pennsylvania. Unfortunately, on day one of our road trip, as we entered Arizona, the Green Queen was not happy. I had never experienced any mechanical issues with my car until that day. However, I also had never driven in 115 degrees. I can't remember how many times we pulled over to let her cool down. When the light-colored steam turned to thick black smoke just outside of Gila Bend, I knew we were done. This was beyond anything we could fix.

As fate would have it, there was someone we knew who lived in Phoenix and could help. My mom and I had both worked for a guy named Bill in San Diego. His brother-in-law, Jim, lived in Phoenix and happened to be great at working on cars. After finding a payphone, we made the call and he agreed to help us. When Jim said that it would take several days, but he was pretty confident he could rebuild the engine, my heart soared with hope. Although my mom was not completely thrilled about this situation, the decision was made that I would stay in Phoenix with the Green Queen and she and Cindy would drive ahead to Missouri, where I would meet them in a week or so. Jim's wife, Nancy, was very kind and agreed to let all of us stay with them that night and for me to extend my stay with them until my car was fixed. Because my mom was not happy about me driving to Missouri by myself, Nancy offered for her cousin, Lyle, to drive with me. I had never met this guy before and was not all that interested in having him as my travel companion. However, who was I to make demands at this point, so I acquiesced. But from that moment on I felt guarded and certain something really bad was going to happen on this trip.

A week later, as my car overheated for what would be the last time, I wondered if my doomsday thoughts had brought this to life. Was this the "really bad thing" that I felt so deeply would happen? Or was this just the fact that the Green Queen was 16 years old and not capable of functioning in this type of heat? As I put on my hazard lights and got out of my car to assess the damage, I realized it really didn't matter. Here we were, in the middle of Arizona, well outside of the city, with no way of communicating for help. If the Green Queen could not recover, we were basically stuck and would have to wait for someone to stop and help us. It was mid-day and the temperature was 121 degrees. We had diet coke and a few snacks with us. We realized quickly that this situation could be quite serious. It was a Wednesday, and this stretch of highway was not populated nor heavily traveled. In fact, when I started thinking about the last time we had passed another vehicle my concern grew. I decided the best thing to do was to get the hood up which might cool off the engine and also let any passersby know the car was disabled.

While I stood in front of my car with Lyle, that doomsday feeling returned. The engine smelled hot and the heat coming up from the highway felt like it was actually melting my flip-flops. One car passed by, and I watched to see if they might pull over to help us, but they kept on going. While I was thinking of options, I thought I heard Lyle say something. I looked over to see what he was saying and realized he was staring at the engine also deep in thought. Then I heard it again, "Get back in the car". The voice was clear like someone was physically speaking to me. Before I realized just what I was doing, I told Lyle we needed to get back in the car. I sat back in my seat and propped my right foot on the center console, trying to get comfortable, knowing that we most likely had a long hot afternoon of waiting ahead of us. Within what had to be less than two minutes, I looked into the rear-view mirror and in the distance saw what I thought was a car coming towards us. The heat coming up off the highway distorted my view, but I could see that there was indeed a car approaching and it was entering the emergency lane. Hooray! Help had arrived! I was about to get out of the car to greet the Good Samaritan, when the same voice, this time much louder said, "stay in the car".

Watching in my rear-view mirror, the heat waves made the car look as though it was moving in slow motion. For just a moment I was mesmerized by the realness and fluidity of the mirage I was seeing. Then my awareness turned back to the car. Something was wrong. The car seemed to be accelerating and was approaching way too fast. I couldn't make sense of what was happening. Why weren't they slowing down? I barely got the words "oh God" out of my mouth before we were rear-ended at a speed of more than 85mph. The sound from the impact was deafening. It felt as though the inside of my car exploded as chards of glass came from every direction. I cringed and held on to the steering wheel as I felt the force of the impact throw me forward. Simultaneously the car lunged forward and to the right sending us down a steep embankment. I wanted to put my foot on the brake, but it was still on the center console. I attempted to pull my leg down, but now there didn't seem to be enough room. It felt like my seat had been pushed forward and I was in this weird bent position. When we finally came to a stop, there was a very strong odor of gasoline. Instinct took over and I knew we needed to get out of the car.

As we stood at the top of the embankment, I had no idea how we had gotten out of the car and were now in this spot. It felt like we had teleported there. I turned to look down at the Green Queen and was completely shocked by what I saw. She was literally half the car she had once been. The rear end was completely folded into what had been the back seat. The back seat was now pushing into the front seats. I was in total disbelief and began shaking uncontrollably feeling as though I was going to collapse. I grabbed onto Lyle's shoulder, so I wouldn't fall. He looked over at me and said, "you're bleeding". I looked down to see multiple streams of blood running down my legs. As I looked up at the sky, I realized I was now lying down. A man with a very bloody face was looking down at me and trying to talk to me but his words were slurred, and I couldn't understand what he was saying. I thought I should get up and help him, but when I tried to, a woman with a very kind voice said, "you need to stay still." I wanted to look up to see her face but couldn't because she was holding my head, so I couldn't turn my neck. I wondered how long she had been here with me. She seemed to know what she was doing so I listened to her.

I could hear bits and pieces of many conversations going on above and around me. Apparently, the man who rear-ended us was drunk because they found open beer cans in his front seat. He had thought my car had been moving, but when he saw the hood up he swerved and as a result hit the driver's side of the rear end of the car. Another man was telling someone that he and his wife had passed us but then heard the impact and came back and were actually the first people to get here. It sounded like a truck driver had been the one to call the police to report the accident. As I listened, I kept seeing the car coming towards us in the rear-view mirror and then going through the crash over and over again. It felt like a movie that was on auto replay and my brain couldn't stop it. Even when I closed my eyes it was still there and running with flashes of the man with the bloody face. It was just too much, and I began to cry. Right now, more than anything, I wished my mom were here. The woman who was holding my head reassured me that everything was going to be ok, and then we heard the sirens in the distance. This time help really was arriving.

After being evaluated at the hospital, I was diagnosed with a concussion and whiplash. Thankfully, Lyle had sustained no injuries and at the time mine seemed to be fairly minor. As we waited for Jim and Nancy to pick us up, I kept thinking about the voice I heard telling me to get in the car and then again to stay there. Had we still been in front of my car when the drunk driver hit us we would have been killed instantly. In my heart I truly believed Divine Intervention had saved our lives. As for the woman at the scene who helped me, it turned out that she had been in the car with her husband and they had passed us just before the accident happened. They had heard the impact, and as a nurse, she felt compelled to come back and help us. Once I was able to talk to my Mom, of course the first thing I wanted her to know was that I was ok. But I also wanted her to know about the voice that saved us. Before I was able to tell her, she told me how she had a premonition about something really bad happening to me and knew I would be in danger. So, the night before my accident she prayed harder than usual and asked God to send a guardian angel to keep me safe. Thanks Mom.

Chapter 2

But Wait, There's More!

"It is difficult to say what is impossible, for the dream of yesterday is the hope of today and the reality of tomorrow. "
–Robert H. Schuller

A s strange as this may sound, June 5th, 1985 will always be a day I celebrate. Yes, that was the day a drunk driver took away my life, as I then knew it, but it could have been the final day listed on my gravestone. Instead, I believe it was the day my true-life journey began. Although it took me quite a while to find my purpose, and it felt like I had way more valleys than peaks during the next twenty years, I began to live my life as a survivor. For the record, that doesn't mean I didn't also live some of those days as a victim, because I did. Especially in the days that immediately followed my accident, I was angry and felt helpless, as victims often do. My whole world had been turned upside down and at nineteen years old I didn't have a plan B. Also, I didn't possess nearly enough life skills needed for what I was about to face.

My first and possibly greatest hurdle was facing my traumatic brain injury, which literally changed almost everything about who I had been. The loss of time and confusion I experienced the day of the accident was given a diagnosis of a concussion. When I was released from the ER, my discharge instructions were very basic. That night someone needed to wake me up every couple of hours and if I started vomiting I should seek additional medical attention. As long as that didn't happen, I should be good to go. Even though I didn't experience any vomiting, I was anything but good to go. In the weeks following my accident I felt confused and sometimes unsure about what exactly had happened. Knowledge I possessed for nearly my entire lifetime now seemed to be distant and out of my reach. Simple things like remembering my social security number took a huge amount of effort to recall. I told myself if I pushed hard enough, I would be ok. There could be nothing further from the truth. The harder I pushed, the more headaches I got and the more difficult it became to put my thoughts together. I began to spiral into an abyss of fear and uncertainty.

Feeling that my family had already been put through enough, I didn't confide in anyone about what I was going through. Instead, I did my best to act as if everything was just fine. In an attempt to regain control, I began writing things down, so I wouldn't forget. I made a list of my social security number, phone number, address and important dates. Even this process became difficult for me. It was as though I could think and see what I wanted to write down, but my hand wouldn't complete the task. And for some strange reason it was also much easier for me to write in all capital letters. Sometimes I would look at what I had written, and it appeared completely foreign to me. I understood that I had written the reminder, but it just wasn't my handwriting anymore. Something else began to occur. I became aware of how much vocabulary I was losing too. Just like the writing, I could see the word I wanted to say, but I sometimes couldn't say the word. Words with multiple syllables were especially difficult. So, I began to replace these words with simpler ones. It felt like I was reverting to my nine-year-old abilities.

When I was nine, I made a list of all the things I would need to accomplish so one day I would be a doctor. There was a lot of education needed to be a doctor and I really liked school, so I thought that part would be pretty easy for me. Doctors had to be able to talk to people about their problems, another thing I enjoyed doing. I was excited when I realized that doctors didn't need to have good handwriting because no matter how much I practiced, and no matter how much Mrs. Wentzel encouraged me, mine just wasn't that terrific. Doctors also had to be able to handle blood and guts, which at the time I secretly thought was super cool. I didn't talk about that with friends because most of them would have found that to be a little creepy. Actually, I didn't talk with my friends about wanting to be a doctor because many of them hadn't a clue what they wanted to be when they grew up, not like I did. At that point in my life I had already been certain for five years. My drive and passion for medicine seemed to have always been with me. I could not remember a time when I wasn't filled with the longing to be a doctor and help people. It simply was part of my DNA.

Somewhere between the car accident and my college orientation, that drive and passion I felt since I was four years old, simply disappeared. Honestly, I didn't even want to go to my college orientation, but my family was so excited about this big event in my life. The last thing I wanted was to be a disappointment to them. I also hoped seeing the campus would help me regain my passion and maybe I could still pull this off. Sadly, the experience left me feeling overwhelmed and more certain than ever that I was not going to be able to attend college. The dream I held in my heart for as long as I could remember was over. This should have been devastating to me, but it wasn't. It actually felt like somewhat of a relief because this dream belonged to a woman I no longer identified with.

In an attempt to regain my identity, I decided to move back to San Diego. It felt like that was the last place where I knew myself. It was also the time during my life when I had everything figured out and my life's purpose was absolutely clear. Currently, I had zero purpose and medical issues that I thought could be better addressed in a larger city like San Diego. So, without a well thought out plan, I flew back to San Diego. This was something my old self would never have done. I had no job and I would be living with a guy I had met a couple of weeks before I left for college and barely knew. As impulsive as that sounds, it made complete sense to the new me.

The new me felt much more spontaneous than the old me. She was carefree and didn't concern herself with plans for the future. She enjoyed living in the moment. She would do whatever she wanted when she wanted. This was so different than the old me who had always tried to please her family and planned to dedicate her life to helping people. The new me didn't really care what anyone thought. The new me seemed the polar opposite of the old me, and she was. Her brain no longer functioned the way it did before. The new me kind of realized she was broken but had no idea how to fix herself. And so, for a while she simply did her best not to think about all she had lost and all that she no longer was.

Before long, the guy she met two weeks before going to college asked her to marry him. Maybe this could be her new life and maybe she could love him enough to be happy as his wife. After all, he had been there for her when she needed someone the most. He didn't love the old her with all the expectations that came with her. He was happy with the simple new her. She didn't want to believe she was settling, but deep inside she knew she was. She also hadn't really paid attention to all the warning signs that existed and should have stopped her from becoming his wife. Their relationship was built on her vulnerability and his love of control. As long as she was weak, he could be strong. As long as she knew her place, he would give her a place beside him. As she began to see glimpses of what her purpose had been and yearned for that once more, she also began to understand the incredible mistake she had made. After only seven months, she knew she had to leave, and so she did.

As my marriage ended, so did my hope of finding my happy ending. Not completely sure if I would ever really return to my original self, I knew I had to learn how to work around the limitations of the new me. This would prove to be nearly impossible. The old me was fearless, but the new me was often paralyzed by fear. Self-doubt and indecision now plagued my thoughts and impacted my daily life. Add extreme impulsivity to the mix and let's just say some days could be a real nightmare. It was the combination of all these things that led to me beginning a new relationship almost immediately following the end of my marriage. At first, this new relationship was passionate and exciting, and I thought maybe I would have my happy ending after all.

After several years of on again and off again, we decided to get married. Once more I ignored the warning signs of this relationship being unhealthy. However, I was truly in love with this man and I wanted a future with him. I believed this relationship was worth fighting for. And, at twenty-seven years old, my clock was ticking, and I wanted to be a mother more than anything else. Somehow, I thought having a baby together would be the ultimate bond that would end any differences between us. Of course, it doesn't work that way, but this child would impact my life in a much more profound way. On the day I gave birth, all the passion and drive I had lost nine years before was restored. The unconditional love I felt for my son ignited a fire in me like I had never felt before. I knew it could never be extinguished by anyone or any event in my life. I also knew my son deserved a mother who was healthy and whole, not broken and divided. From this point on, there would be no old me and new me. The only me that mattered would be the Mom-me.

Chapter 3

Puzzle Pieces

"Hope rises like a phoenix from the ashes of shattered dreams."
–S.A. Sachs

F or as long as I had dreamed of becoming a doctor, I also dreamed of becoming a mom. Although I always envisioned motherhood happening after becoming a doctor, it was never second in any way. The plan was to go to school, get my medical degree, get married and then start a family. In my mind, that seemed simple and straightforward. Because I was the ultimate planner, I had even thought about the age I would be when I gave birth. The age I figured would be just about perfect was twenty-eight. With all the life events that did not go as planned, becoming a mom at twenty-eight was the one thing that had. As if that wasn't amazing enough, the healing that followed was an unexpected gift. The metamorphosis into motherhood ignited both the strength and determination that had left me nearly a decade before.

As I began facing new hurdles and possibly some of my darkest hours, I leaned into this strength and determination to push through. Before my son's first birthday, my second marriage would end, adding another failure to my already list of many (more about that later). The ideal life I wanted for my son was nowhere in sight. We were left homeless and had no choice but to move in with my Dad and his wife, Niki. Although I will always be grateful to them for giving us a roof over our heads, I don't think any of us imagined this scenario or rejoiced in its occurrence. I think it is only fair to say that we all made the best of a rather tough situation. So here I was, divorced for the second time, without a place to call my own and navigating single parenthood the best I possibly could.

Realizing I needed to do much better, I sought out a counselor who might be able to help me wrap my head around my head. When I walked into her office for the first time she told me her name was Carol. Her swollen belly told me she must be in the last trimester of her pregnancy. This circumstance instantly connected us. I was a first-time mom and she was about to be. Carol wanted to make sure I would be ok with our rather short time period to work together. After assuring her I thought eight weeks would be enough time, we dug right in. When she asked what had brought me here, I told her it was my son. I was here because I wanted him to have a healthy, happy mom. My child deserved the best possible version of me.

During my weekly sessions with Carol, I began to feel like myself again. I was starting to see glimpses of the woman I knew and understood. Through truly feeling my emotions I was able to let go of the past and find clarity about my future. Carol encouraged me to "own" my feelings, no matter what they were. If I felt angry, then I should express my anger. If I felt sadness, I should let the tears flow. I hadn't realized the gigantic wall I had built to keep my emotions in check. Carol also helped me to see that the unconditional love I feel for my son should be a gift I give to myself, as well. This was a complete game changer for me. The unconditional love I felt for Anthony was always abundant and always present. All I had to do was think about him and I was immediately filled with it.

For the next two and a half years, I focused on this love and being the absolute best mom I could be. Nothing came before Anthony. Every decision I made was based on his best interest. There was an enormous amount of friction with my ex-husband about custody and visitation. Each time I had to endure another court proceeding, I drew strength from the unconditional love I felt for my son. With all my sincerity I wanted nothing more than for my ex-husband to have a healthy relationship with his son. However, I soon had to face the realization my son's welfare included limiting the exposure to his biological father. He had serious anger management issues, which were made worse by substance abuse. To keep Anthony safe from this behavior, I asked for a court order to have my ex-husband drug tested if I suspected use before or during his visitation. If he refused to test, or tested positive, I had the right to withhold visitation. Thankfully, the court granted me this order.

Shortly after Anthony and I moved into our own place, my sister Korey asked me if I would ever think about dating again. My response was immediate. The only man I wanted in my life was

Anthony. I didn't want to date anyone and certainly didn't want to introduce some strange guy to my kid. My focus was strictly on being a good mom. However, that conversation began to make me think about the need for a healthy male role model for my son. For the first time in my life though, I was not thinking about a man in a romantic way. I just wanted a great guy friend to hang out with who would be a good role model for Anthony. Great idea, but how does a single mom meet such a person? My resourceful sister knew exactly how to make this happen.

Before I had a chance to change my mind, Korey brought over a computer and had me signed up with America Online (AOL). She told me all about these chat rooms where single parents could be friends and get to know each other. I still don't know for certain, but I suspect this was her idea of how to warm me up to start dating again. Kind of like a blind date, but much sneakier. And believe me, Korey is one of the sneakiest little sisters on the planet. In fact, her sneaking around when we were kids resulted in her finding all the gifts that Santa was supposed to bring us. Which in turn proved there was no Santa. I was devastated. This time though, I think her sneakiness came from a genuine place of love and the wish for her big sister to be happy. This wish would end up giving me one of the greatest gifts I could ever ask for.

Turns out the single parenting chat room was full of people who wanted to find other single parents to date. Which was exactly the opposite thing I was interested in. So, I turned off the computer and went to bed. A few nights later, I decided to try again. I began looking at all the different chat room names and rolled my eyes as I read their ridiculous titles. I was about to turn off my computer when a chat room called "The nicest guy on AOL" caught my eye. Seriously, I thought to myself, who thought of this name? As I entered the room, I saw the screen name "eyestwinkle", immediately thought of Santa Claus and smiled. So, I thought what the heck and read the profile attached to the screen name. The name listed was Todd and he lived in Denver, CO. At the bottom was an area for a favorite quote. His was "I would rather believe in the dream she is out there, than the nightmare she isn't." As I read this, something inside me stirred. I understood the feeling of the hope and of the sadness this quote held.

This was the first time I had reached out to anyone in a chat room. My bravery was boosted a bit by the fact he lived in Denver. The risk seemed minimal and so I typed my first question. "Are you the nicest guy on AOL?" He responded, "No, I'm the second nicest." That made me smile again. I thought that was a good response and liked his sense of humor. So, I asked another question. "Are you Santa Clause?" He said, "nope, just one of the elves." That response made me giggle. And that is exactly how our friendship began. We began to meet online each evening after Anthony was tucked in and asleep for the night. It was a wonderful arrangement and I soon found myself looking forward to our evening exchanges. After a month or so, Todd asked if we could talk on the phone. This was 1997 and Caller ID was still not widely used, so I thought it would be safe for me to call him. There was no way I was giving out any of my personal information to him. Especially since my friend Anna kept reminding me he was most likely a serial killer.

When he answered the phone, his voice was friendly, and I remember feeling very relaxed almost immediately. Our conversation was easy and familiar, as if two old friends were catching up. We had typed about so many things but talking to one another seemed to fill in all the details. As I listened to him tell me about his life, the more I wanted to know this man. Without a doubt we had a genuine connection. There was no secret agenda or pressure for this to be anything more than it was. We were just two human beings getting to know each other. Looking back, I think we both may have needed this time more than we knew. Both of us had been in long-term relationships that ended in divorce. Neither of us had expected to be single again at this stage in our lives.

After nearly four months of typing and talking we agreed it was time to meet. Because Anna was still not convinced Todd wasn't a serial killer, we agreed he would come to San Diego for our first meeting. On October 3rd, 1997 that day finally arrived. I was so excited to meet this man who I had a deep connection and friendship with. Was I hoping for it to be more than a friendship at some point? I would be a liar if I didn't admit that I was hoping for more. What I was not prepared for was experiencing something I thought was impossible. When our eyes met for the first time, it was truly love at first sight.

Chapter 4

Blended By Love

"Love recognizes no barriers. It jumps hurdles, leaps fences,
penetrates walls to arrive at its destination full of hope"
–Maya Angelou

F rom the moment Todd and I met we knew we were soul mates. Neither of us had ever felt this way about anyone else before. The fact that this relationship had been built on friendship only made it more special. It wasn't a matter of if we would get married, but when. The first step would be finding a way to live closer to one another. When we looked at the big picture, it made more sense for me to relocate. An added bonus was that I could work remotely. Which meant Anthony would no longer have to be in daycare. However, this included going back to court to ask for permission to leave San Diego with Anthony. My plan also included having my mom move to Denver to help me in case I needed to travel for work.

Fast-forward to May of 1998. The planets have aligned and Anthony and I, just as we had planned, are now living in Denver. My mom arrived shortly after us. There were now three generations of my family living under one roof. Hooray for Anthony! He has his mom, grandma and his "Toddy" all loving and supporting him every day. Not to mention his new big boy racecar bed. Life is good. This new beginning could not be any better. My relationship with Todd strengthens with each passing day. He also has great rapport with my mom. But it is Todd's relationship with Anthony that is beyond amazing. This wonderful man has taken on this little boy as if he were his own child. My wish for Anthony to have a positive male role model in his life has come true.

Just a few months later, as we all were settling into our routines, my mom received a call from my grandpa. He was struggling with caring for my Aunt Pat. She was my mom's older sister and was born with fairly significant developmental delays. Pat also struggled with Parkinson's disease. She had always lived at home with my grandparents. My grandma Dorothy, who was Pat's primary care giver, had passed right before I met Todd. She was only seventy-five and her death had been unexpected. My grandpa was doing his best to care for Pat, but their relationship was becoming strained. He asked my mom if she could move back to Pennsylvania to help. We all understood what her answer needed to be.

With my mom headed back to Pennsylvania, it would have been so easy for Anthony and I to move in with Todd. But I felt strongly that living together would not be best for us. I wanted the commitment of marriage before we took that step. I had lived with both of my husbands before getting married. Looking back, it felt like that had been a mistake. This time I also had a child's heart to consider. So, I stood my ground and moved into a smaller apartment that was perfect for Anthony and I. We spent a lot of time together with Todd, but at the end of the day, we both had our separate households. This boundary felt very healthy to me.

My little boy had a different idea of what he wanted. Anthony began to ask why he couldn't call Todd "daddy". He thought having two daddies was better than having one. He also couldn't understand why Toddy wasn't with us all the time. There didn't seem like an easy way of explaining all of this to a four-year-old. Instead, I focused on our love for one another. We talked about how people who love each other can be apart and the love doesn't go away. Even though we aren't physically together, the love stays in our hearts. Anthony seemed to be satisfied with this explanation. I hoped before he asked more questions that were difficult to answer Todd would be ready to move forward.

On May 26th, 2000, while we were on vacation in Pennsylvania visiting my family, Todd proposed. We had the best day as a family at Knoebel's Grove, a local amusement park where I used to go to as a kid. It was so fun sharing this with Todd and Anthony, making new memories with them. My grandpa, mom and aunt all went along that day. The day had been simply perfect. That night Anthony was staying with my mom, so Todd and I could have some alone time. Later that night he asked me to go for a walk. I had no idea what was about to happen. We eventually stopped in front of my grandparent's old house, a place where I had so many fond childhood memories. He knew this place was very dear to my heart and would be the perfect spot to ask me to marry him. I said yes!

In December of that same year, I came up with this crazy idea to have a surprise wedding on New Year's Eve. Why spend money on a big wedding, when we could have an intimate one in our own home? Anthony was six years old and he thought surprises were awesome. He loved the idea of keeping this a secret. So, in three weeks we made all the arrangements and invited our guests for a New Year's Eve party. We told our families we wanted them present but also understood this might not be possible given the timeline. They opted to be present by phone. At 11pm our best man Matthew, announced to all our guests they were taking part in an elaborate ruse. They had actually been invited to a wedding. Todd and I exchanged vows as husband and wife and added special vows to include Anthony. At the stroke of midnight on 01/01/01 we officially became the Felts Family.

The rest of this year turned out to be one of our best for making memories, and one of our toughest for facing heartbreaking moments. The next big event was my dear friend Anna getting married to her fiancé Eli. Anna was Anthony's godmother and she had been there for us during some really tough times. They planned to have a romantic wedding in Charleston on May 19th and asked Anthony and I to be part of it. We decided to plan our honeymoon around this event. Knowing we wanted Anthony to go with us, our itinerary would include Disney World, Animal Kingdom, Kennedy Space Center and end with a Disney Cruise to the Bahamas. As if that wasn't enough, when we got home from our trip we rescued our first dog, Bailey the Beagle. What an amazing first six months our family had!

Todd and I knew we wanted more children and began trying to get pregnant as soon as we returned from our trip. Anthony really wanted to be a big brother and continually asked us when that would happen. In August, we succeeded and were over the moon. We decided to surprise Anthony with this news on September 19th, his 7th birthday. On September 11th, our world was turned upside down. Our future suddenly felt uncertain as our nation faced the ramification of this terrorist attack. For our son and unborn child, Todd and I both felt we must get back to normalcy as soon as possible. We could not let this event paralyze us. No matter what the future held, we decided the Felts Family would not buckle.

We had a pirate party for Anthony's 7th birthday and invited all our neighbors and their kids. For a few hours we were all pirates and fully enveloped in walking the plank and searching for buried treasure. It felt good to see our friends and their kids enjoying themselves. For a few hours, life seemed normal again and that was such a gift. The best gift was wrapping up a tiny pair of baby booties and giving them to Anthony. When he opened the box and saw what was inside his face filled with joy. We didn't have to explain. Anthony understood he was going to be a big brother.

As September ended and October began, our family was so full of hope for the future. Although our world was now unpredictable in so many ways, our family unit felt secure. Soon there would be another member of the Felts family. A special child would be born and fully connect our blended family. When Todd came home on October 10th and told me had been laid off, I did my best not to be shaken. His company had decided to move tech support to India and his position was now obsolete. I was working full time and made enough to support our family. We would be ok.

Less than a month after Todd lost his job, my worst nightmare began. I started spotting. I thought, no, this couldn't be happening, not again. Most doctors say spotting during pregnancy can be normal for some women. In my heart, I knew this wasn't normal for me. I had experienced this before and it ended in miscarriage. Within twenty-four hours the spotting turned to heavy bleeding. My doctor confirmed there was no longer a heartbeat. Todd and I were heart broken. The heart we worried most about though was Anthony's. Telling our little boy that he wasn't going to be a big brother after all nearly tore our hearts apart.

Although we continued to try, Todd and I were not able to have any more children. Anthony would never be a big brother. Our dream of having a large family together would not come to fruition. This could have taken such a toll on our family. Instead, we chose to celebrate the gift we had already been given. Nearly all of us are born into this world with no choice in the matter. Anthony was not Todd's biological child, but he had chosen him to be his Daddy. That choice, and the unconditional love of a child, was all we needed to blend our family.

Chapter 5

I Surrender

"The very least you can do in your life is figure out what you hope for. And the most you can do is live inside that hope. Not admire it from a distance but live right in it, under its roof."
–Barbara Kingsolvery

As we settled into the normalcy of being a family and our daily schedules, work and homework filled our days. Movies, pizza and sleepovers filled our nights. Life was simple and easy. Anthony was a typical ten-year-old hanging out with his friends. Todd and I were settling into an ordinary life as a married couple. I cannot tell you how good simple and ordinary felt. Although I was not fulfilled in my work life, my home life more than made up for it. I was happy with my life. Todd and Anthony were all I needed.

One Saturday, which seemed no different than any other Saturday, our lives took a dramatic turn. Todd came home from running errands and was acting oddly. At first, I thought he had been drinking and was more than a little annoyed with him. I had zero tolerance for drinking and driving and he knew that. Fairly quickly I realized he was not drunk. He attempted to tell me he had lost his peripheral vision, but his words were slurred and jumbled. The look in his eyes was a mixture of confusion and fear. Something was very wrong.

As we raced to the hospital, because Todd refused to let me call 911, I was hoping we'd get there in time. As soon as we arrived, Todd was rushed into the ER. They believed, as I did, he was having a stroke. Watching my husband be unable to communicate and seeing the fear in his eyes tore me up. But I knew I had to be strong and communicate for him. Something inside me awakened, pushing my fear away and allowing me to give a concise report to the medical team. I was able to share his symptoms and time of onset. It was exactly what they needed in order to help Todd.

After what seemed like an eternity, the doctor came in to talk with us. Fortunately, they determined Todd did not have a stroke. However, the diagnosis was still concerning. They believed Todd had experienced a complex migraine. Due to the significant neurological symptoms exhibited, he needed to follow up with his regular doctor for more testing as soon as possible. It was important to determine the origin, what caused this event. We left the hospital feeling grateful and yet very uncertain, once again, about what the future held.

Within a few weeks Todd was referred to a neurosurgeon. After reviewing his MRI, the doctor told us how fortunate it was Todd had a complex migraine. If it were not for that situation, Todd would be walking around undiagnosed with a much more serious health issue, which could dramatically change his life forever. The MRI revealed moderate spinal cord impingement, making him an immediate surgical candidate. Had he taken a fall, and landed just the right way, he would have become a paraplegic instantly.

In January of 2005, as soon as we had authorization from our insurance company, Todd was scheduled for surgery at Sky Ridge Medical Center. This event would not only change Todd's life, but mine as well. We were fortunate to have many amazing nurses after his surgery, but one in particular went above and beyond. Cindy was competent, kind and really understood how to connect with her patients. She also understood the importance of connecting with the patient's family. Our connection led us to a conversation about my plans to become a nurse. Something I had been thinking about for several years but never acted on. I certainly had never talked about it with people I barely knew. But something about Cindy made me feel like I could, like I wanted to. She even offered to be a reference for me if I decided to apply at Sky Ridge. When it was time for Todd to discharge, we exchanged contact information and I told her I would call her once I decided what I was going to do.

During the last week of April, my grandpa and I talked on the phone like we did most Saturdays. This conversation was like many we had, talking about the weather, as we were both huge weather enthusiasts. He had been teaching me about the weather since I was a kid. The topics we talked about never really mattered. It was more about hearing each other's voices. He may have needed that, but I know I always needed it more. Hearing his voice and being in his presence had always made me feel safe. He was gentle and kind and only on a very rare occasion stern with me.

During this conversation his tone felt kind of stern. He wanted to know about my plans for nursing school. As I tried to explain that I couldn't possibly think about that right now because Anthony and Todd needed me, he wouldn't have it. He then revealed something I never knew. He told me my grandma Dorothy had always wanted to be a nurse. She had said the same things to him that I was now saying. He always wanted to give her the world and yet this is the one thing he never supported her on. It was a regret he would not allow to be repeated. He made me promise him that I would become a nurse.

The following Saturday, we didn't get to talk because he wasn't feeling that great. One week later, my grandpa passed from pneumonia. Had he known he was going to pass? Is that why he was so insistent about telling me about my grandma Dorothy? I may never know the answer to those questions, but I do know this: he spent his last days telling everyone he knew his granddaughter was going to nursing school. At his funeral and afterwards I was asked several times "Are you the granddaughter that's going to be a nurse?" As soon as we got back to Colorado, I gave my two week notice and applied for CNA School. It was the beginning of my path to keep my promise to my Grandpa.

As soon as I graduated from CNA School, I reached out to Cindy. She was more than willing to put in a good word for me with Sky Ridge. I have no doubt Vicky, the department head of the Med/Surg, would not have agreed to meet with me otherwise.

During our interview she struggled with the fact I had left a much higher paying job and was now applying for a position that only paid nearly half of my previous one. Somehow, my passion came through and she agreed to hire me. My connection with Cindy led me to this opportunity with Vicky. I will be forever grateful to both of these women for seeing the potential nurse in me. It is a constant reminder for me to do the same for others that cross my path.

I have had the honor of working with many amazing nurses over the years, but none have had as great an impact on me as the nurses at Sky Ridge. When I started on nightshift, Susan and Kathy were both very experienced Med/Surg nurses who took me under their wings. Susan was a combination of Mother Teresa mixed with your favorite standup comedian. She taught me the importance of having both faith and fun. Kathy had been a nurse for as long as nursing certificates had been given out. Her years of experience in Med/Surg made her the expert in any situation. Yet she didn't crave moving on from being a floor nurse. She taught me about finding your lane and staying in it if it made you happy. A banana Popsicle near the end of each shift made Kathy very happy. I often searched many a hospital freezer to bring her this little piece of happiness.

When I moved to day shift a whole new world opened up for me. The group of day shift nurses on the 6th floor was a force to be reckoned with. They were fiercely loyal to one another and always willing to help each other out when it hit the fan as it often did. Jenn was the epitome of what an ethical nurse acted like. She taught me to never consider crossing the line, no matter how small, no matter what. Jeanne was so competent and capable. She helped me understand the importance of always using critical thinking.

Ashley was young and a brand-new nurse who shined with promise. She taught me to always keep that brand-new nurse shine. Glenda was the nurse every other nurse and patient loved. Glenda the good nurse taught me to always be kind. Anna was our charge nurse on most days. She could be tough, but she was always fair. She taught me that being a leader wasn't always easy, but you still needed to step up and lead. Carol was the nurse you were always glad to see on the schedule. She never created drama or made any situation about her. She taught me to keep my head down and to roll with the punches.

Sometimes you meet people who you just click with and know you want to be in your life. Misty is one of these people and a spectacular nurse. We were blessed to have Misty care for Todd after his second neck surgery. During this time, she listened to my concerns about Todd's breathing. She took the time to stay and watch him breathe. Turned out Todd had significant sleep apnea. Misty taught me about the importance of always making time, listening and taking action to help your patient.

There are spectacular nurses and then there are superstar nurses. Jill and Sharon were definitely in this second category. They were part of our super flex pool team. Which meant each of them had to be proficient in at least four nursing specialties. Although they were experts, they were two of those most compassionate nurses I have ever met. Both of them taught me to always give 100% to each of my patients. No matter what the outcome may be, you can look back and know you gave that patient your best. And if ever you felt like you couldn't do that anymore, you had no business being a nurse. That passion for helping people will never leave me.

It was during this time, surrounded by all these amazing nurses, I was finally able to let go. I wasn't giving into a "plan b" for my life. I was finally accepting what my life was intended to be. I surrendered and stopped resisting my true path. Some people consider surrendering as admitting defeat. I totally disagree. I surrendered to leaving the broken past behind me, which is anything but defeat. The act of surrender gave me the freedom to be the healer I was always meant to be.

Chapter 6

The Power of
Human Connection

"A new baby is like the beginning of all things—
wonder, hope, a dream of possibilities."
–Eda J LeShan

From the moment of conception and for nearly the first year of our life while in utero, we share an extraordinary human connection with our mother. Studies show this connection is both biological and psychological, and experienced on a mutual level. Ask any woman who has been pregnant, and she will tell you she doesn't need a study to confirm this. Increasing levels of estrogen and progesterone create changes in her body that are necessary for a healthy pregnancy. The rise in hormones cause side effects that have the ability to alter her mood, sense of taste, sense of smell and even her eyesight. Some women endure what seems like endless days of vomiting and exhaustion during the early part of their pregnancy. Yet other women may not experience any of these negative side effects.

Something that does seem to be nearly universal for first time pregnant women is wondering if she will be a good mom and worrying about her baby being born healthy. There doesn't seem to be any amount of reassurance that can be offered to stop these thoughts. Of course, these thoughts can cause stress and one of the first things pregnant women are told is to reduce daily stress because it will affect their baby. Basically, the message is that happy healthy moms have happy healthy babies. Which seems simple enough, until she starts adding in a few dynamics that sometimes occur in a less than perfect life. Maybe she still needs to work full time during her pregnancy whether she has the energy to or not. Maybe this pregnancy was not planned and now she's trying to figure out how it fits into her life. Maybe this pregnancy is the product of a less than perfect marriage. The list goes on and on.

In 1994, my list began with working full time and being in a less than perfect marriage. But the item on the list most impacting this pregnancy was the fact that my last pregnancy had ended in a miscarriage. My doctor told me it was not uncommon to have a miscarriage before carrying a pregnancy to full term. He explained that a miscarriage usually happens because something is wrong with the embryo. He told me not to worry because I was young and still had plenty of time to have as many babies as I wanted. But in that moment, I wasn't thinking about other babies because

I was very sad about the loss of this baby. Even though it was very early in my pregnancy I was devastated. What made it worse was the feeling that my husband wasn't nearly as disappointed as I was.

Although it took me well over a year to get pregnant again, this pregnancy felt completely different from my last one. Almost immediately, very intense nausea and vomiting began. My morning sickness was more like all day sickness, but I looked at it as a sign that my hormones must be high, and it meant my pregnancy was viable. When I made it through my first trimester with no signs of any trouble, I finally began to relax a little bit. Just a few weeks later, I felt my baby move for the first time. My mom had told me it kind of felt like a butterfly fluttering. I could not have described the physical feeling any better, but there really are no words to convey the joy of that moment. It was the first time I experienced being connected to my baby and the first time I felt the unconditional love that comes with that.

When I found out I was going to have a son I was so surprised, because for some reason I thought I was having a girl. In fact, I had already chosen her name and had been calling her Claire. After apologizing to him for this innocent mistake, I quickly became very excited to meet my little man. I talked to him endlessly about all we would do when he was born. I explained that I had waited so long to be his mom and that had just given me more time to build my love for him. There would never be another boy loved as much as he would be loved. I also gave him my word that I would always protect him and keep him safe. I promised him that he would always be able to count on me no matter what.

When Anthony was just eight months old, I kept that promise. It was my first Mother's Day and after an altercation that could have ended with Anthony being significantly harmed, the future became very clear. For years, I hadn't been able to find enough value in myself to believe I deserved better, but I absolutely knew Anthony did. The unconditional love and connection I had with my son gave me the strength I needed to do for him what I could not do for myself and finally leave my abusive marriage. On my second Mother's Day, having had time to heal and reflect, I came to the realization that while I may have had a part in giving Anthony life, he had a bigger part in saving mine. Thank you, Boy.

Twelve years later, when I started nursing school, I was leaning towards becoming a labor and delivery nurse. Because of the positive impact Anthony's birth had on my life, I thought being able to share that with other moms would be amazing. During my "Mom Baby" rotation, as a student nurse at Aurora Medical Center, I was fortunate to be paired with a nurse who had been helping deliver babies for over twenty years. It was so easy to see that she absolutely loved what she was doing. And, even though she had been a nurse for more than twenty years, she told me she could still remember how overwhelming it was to be a nursing student. She was kind and encouraging and helped bolster my confidence. At the end of my rotation, with her supervision, I was able to assist in my first delivery.

During our report we were told this was the mother's first pregnancy. She was in her early twenties and already having contractions when she arrived at the hospital. Fear and pain were evident in her eyes as my preceptor and I entered her room. I quickly realized that she only spoke and understood a small amount of English. Her husband and family were with her for support. He was bilingual and able to help translate as we asked her questions and explained what we were doing to prepare her for delivery.

Initially, I allowed my biggest enemy, self-doubt, to invade me. Will I be able to start the IV? Will I remember the position for the fetal monitor to be placed? What if I can't communicate with her? How will I help her deliver this baby if she can't understand what I'm saying? And then it happened. I stopped worrying about all these "what ifs" and just simply focused on our human connection. Our eyes met, and I smiled. When she smiled back, I reached for her hand and gently squeezed it. She squeezed back. That simple connection made me feel less doubtful. I began to believe I could do this. I began to feel hopeful.

As her labor progressed, we continued our connection. I began to feel connected to her husband and family. Even though I wasn't able to fully communicate with words, I focused on making eye contact, smiling and at times placing my hand on each family member's shoulder. From time to time, the family would ask the husband to translate their appreciation to me. I would smile and nod my head signaling my gratitude for their appreciation, never speaking a word of Spanish.

My preceptor continued to check-in to monitor the progression of labor and make sure I was doing ok. She made me feel safe and supported as she validated my clinical reports. Clearly, she was giving me the opportunity to build confidence in a caring and supportive environment. She not only gave me the opportunity to be involved with this birth but understood that I needed to be an active participant, as well.

Several hours later, near the end of my shift, a beautiful healthy baby girl entered this world. The moment held a mixture of tears, laughter, excitement, and relief for this new mom and dad and their family. As I watched in amazement, the labor and delivery team interacted with one another as if they had done this a million times, each knowing their specific role and performing it without hesitation. All the while, they were cooing over the baby and reassuring the new parents in the process. I stood back and took in all that was happening medically, as a good nursing student should; I glanced down at the baby and it was as if nothing else in the room mattered anymore. The crying and kicking had stopped. She lay on her back with her head tilted towards me with the most perfectly serene expression on her face.

As I met her gaze, trying to remember the distance at which newborns could see, I felt compelled to go to her. When I was about two feet away, one of the nurses approached and I stopped, realizing I might be getting too close. Instead of telling me not to get any closer, she smiled and said, "it's ok, she won't break". I smiled nervously and continued toward the baby. I knelt down, my face about twelve inches from hers and once again met her gaze. Quite simply, I was awestruck. I felt an overwhelming feeling of joy. So much so, I felt tears welling up in my eyes. My preceptor came to stand next to me, putting her hand on my shoulder. She said, "pretty amazing, huh?" I couldn't speak, just nodded, but she understood. In that profound moment, I understood the power of human connection, and how witnessing a birth connects our lives forever. It wasn't until later in my career that I would come to realize the significance of human connection as the genesis of hope.

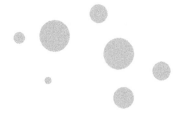

Chapter 7

Eating Their Young

"I find hope in the darkest of days and focus
in the brightest. I do not judge the universe."
–Dalai Lama

I n nursing we have this motto "See one, do one, teach one".
Sounds easy enough, but it's often not realized because of
another less attractive phenomenon that exists in the field
of Nursing. Unfortunately, all too often experienced nurses who
precept student nurses or new nurses feel like they have to be
really tough on them. It's known as "eating their young". During
clinical rotations, I had the displeasure of being in the company
of one such nurse. It was as if beating down nursing students was
her favorite way to pass the time. I imagine that she too had been

beaten down when she was a student and felt as though this was some type of hazing ritual that all nurses go through to earn their nursing pin.

One of her very creative ways to instill fear in her students was to ask each of us the same question on the very first day of our assignment. "What are you afraid of?" Sounds innocent doesn't it? However, as we went around the table spilling our guts, she would challenge our answers. If she felt the fear was not warranted she would ask again. "What are you REALLY afraid of?" When it was my turn to answer, my initial thought was, you. You scare me. But instead I replied, "I don't want to make a mistake that could seriously harm someone". What I didn't know then was how much she would use these fears against us during our rotation with her. At almost every turn she would point out something done wrong. Even if 9 out of the 10 steps to a process were done correctly, she would focus on the one that was incorrect. We all dreaded going to this clinical site because of it. We all vowed that if we stuck together (safety in numbers) we could get through this. That vow would end up giving me hope during one of the most hopeless times in my life.

At the halfway point of the rotation, my son was diagnosed with a serious illness that would require care at Children's Hospital. A few days later, my husband received devastating news that his 50-year-old brother Scott had suddenly died. Needless to say, it would have been a very difficult time without the added stress of being a nursing student. However, I was determined to make it through this clinical while still putting my family first. Unfortunately, there was another hurdle just ahead of me, nearly ending my nursing career before it even started.

My nursing school had a very stringent attendance policy that included both the classroom and clinical rotation portions of our education. The only way to miss any clinical time was by making arrangements with your clinical instructor to make-up the missed hours. If your clinical instructor was not willing to do this or felt the reason for your absence was not warranted, you could be placed on clinical probation. Up until now, my attendance had been perfect. As you can probably imagine, I was extremely hesitant about approaching this particular clinical instructor. However, given the circumstances, I also felt fairly confident that my circumstances warranted being able to miss a day or two.

A few days later, during my evaluation with my instructor, I requested time off from my rotation to attend my brother-in-law's funeral. We also discussed my son's recent diagnosis and options for treatment. Quite honestly, I hoped that disclosing these personal details of my life with her might spark a human connection and lend her to be empathetic about my predicament and work with me. Instead, she used the opportunity to tell me that it was going to be nearly impossible to make up my hours; she had serious doubts about my clinical skills, thought I had a poor attitude and wasn't applying myself.

While the exact words spoken are not memorable, the feeling of being at her mercy while she berated me still conjures a visceral reaction in me to this day. It was one of the most paralyzing moments of my life as someone in a position of power completely dominated me and ruthlessly took advantage of my extreme vulnerability. As self-doubt spread through my mind, I began to second-guess everything I had accomplished until now as a nursing student. Just as I thought I could take no more the survivor in me screamed, "FIGHT". And fight I did. My words were precise, my voice was steady, my message was clear. I told her she was wrong about me. This person she assumed I was could not be further from the truth. My dedication and intention were 100% intact. My sole purpose for becoming a nurse was to make a difference and through previous patient and clinical instructor comments I knew I was on my way to doing just that. However, during this clinical rotation something was different. I told her I believed the difference was the instructor. She instilled fear, not confidence. She focused on weaknesses rather than strengths. She made all criticism personal rather than constructive. I concluded by telling her I accepted I couldn't miss any time for my brother-in-law's funeral and would not ask for any time off for my son's health issues either. I also stated that it would probably be a good idea for her and I to meet with my school to work through any further unresolved matters. She said that wouldn't be necessary and would turn in my evaluation directly to the school. As I left the clinical site that day I vowed not to be alone with this person ever again; a vow that was made a little too late.

The next day, I received a call from the Dean of my school, asking me to come in to discuss an urgent matter. As I entered his office, he and the Director of Nursing, Carol were sitting down waiting for me. The expression on both their faces was grave. This was definitely not a good sign. I was told that I couldn't finish my clinical rotation because the instructor felt I was unsafe. I knew there had been friction between us, but I had no idea she would go so far as to ban me from coming back to my rotation and accuse me of unsafe practices. However, when I began to read the litany of alleged incidents that she claimed occurred I quickly realized this was a personal vendetta to make me pay for having spoken up during our last interaction. As I continued to read the list of exaggerations and complete un-truths, the Dean told me that this potentially constituted my being removed from the nursing program. To say I was devastated does not even begin to describe my emotions.

The situation seemed completely hopeless. She had won. She was in a position of power and it was her word against mine. All I had worked so hard for, all that I had given up, all that I had asked my family to give up, it was all gone. As the immensity of the moment overwhelmed me, the tears I had been holding back for quite some time began to flow and in that moment, I felt more hopeless and alone than I think I ever had in my life. And then it happened. The out reached hand of the Director of Nursing came into my tear-filled vision, offering me a tissue and asking for my side of the story.

As my voice trembled and a myriad of emotions flooded my mind, I nodded my head and attempted to gather my thoughts. My first inclination was to defend myself and tell them both that this lady hated me. But then I thought, how would that sound? Like a guilty kid trying to get out of her punishment. No, I needed to make sure they knew all the facts without being defensive. They both knew me. Knew I was passionate about being a nurse. They knew how much my family and I had given up being accepted to this nursing program. They also knew that I was a dedicated student who often stood up and challenged things if I thought it was in the best interest of a patient or fellow student. Including challenging a test or two where over half my class had failed. They may have even thought I was outspoken at times. But they knew me. They knew the horrible things that this instructor accused me of were out of character. Thankful for our previous interactions and the human connection we had, I made the most of the opportunity they were giving me.

My active participation in this moment included explaining different scenarios and answering their questions. Encouraging them to speak with the other students in this rotation with me to get their perception of my behavior, participation and that of the instructor. My success at previous clinical sites was discussed and suggestions were made to interview those clinical instructors. Most important, I accepted responsibility for my part in all of this. Although I felt I had to stand up for myself at the time, and was under a tremendous amount of emotional stress, if I had it to do over again, I would not challenge this person. Even if what she said truly hurt me, because nothing would hurt me as much as losing the opportunity to become a nurse and disappoint my family in the process.

As I left the Dean's office I felt completely spent both physically and emotionally, yet strangely hopeful. The case for my future was pled through honesty and humility. My passion and desire to be a nurse was undeniable. I had listened and been listened to. My connection with these two faculty members had strengthened because of this interaction. I prayed they would find me innocent of any wrongdoing and allow me to stay in the program, because I truly feared I would lose my mind if they did not.

The next forty-eight hours were brutal. While my class continued their clinical rotations, I was sidelined spending much of my waking hours ruminating nearly to the point of insanity.

During the investigation I was instructed not to speak with any of my classmates. If word got back to the faculty that I had, it would mean immediate expulsion. I confided in my family and was grateful for their support. However, I felt guilty for adding this burden to my husband's already full plate of grief after just receiving the news his brother had died. And so, I turned to someone whom I had quickly become close to in school. Although she was a fellow student, I knew I could trust her to keep my confidence.

Not only did Gretchen keep my confidence, she restored it, as well. She gave me the opportunity to tell my story and grieve my mistakes, over and over again. She listened patiently without casting any judgment on my actions or me. She had faith in my abilities as a nursing student and kept reminding me of that truth as I began the endless cycle of self-doubt. At one point, she told me that she would go to the Dean on my behalf and plead my case. And, if that weren't enough she would start a petition. She was absolutely, 100% on my side and her friendship never wavered. In many ways, she was a catalyst for my theory of H+O+P=E. It was my connection with her that kept me hopeful during this tumultuous time and through all the remaining ups and downs of nursing school.

When the call came in from the school that the allegations were unfounded, and my name had been cleared, my initial reaction was that of relief and thankfulness. Soon after, I started to wonder how many other students this person had negatively affected. I was determined to be an advocate for any student who was encountering this type of treatment by an instructor.

Imagine my surprise when I found out that my school was no longer going to use this particular person as a clinical instructor as a result of my investigation and testimony. Strike one up for the nursing students!

Chapter 8

Opportunity Knocks

"Learn from yesterday, live for today, hope for tomorrow.
The important thing is not to stop questioning."
–Albert Einstein

A s one door closed in my clinical rotation, another opened. This particular door would have a huge impact on my nursing career. Because I had to complete my clinical rotation at another facility, my Psychiatric Nursing clinical had to be changed to a different facility too. I ended up at Fort Logan, the State of Colorado mental health facility. Some fellow nursing students considered this a fate almost worse than death. Well, maybe not worse than death but certainly worse than any other clinical site my school had to offer for psychiatric rotation.

After what I had just endured, I really wasn't too concerned about it being that bad. Plus, there were rumors about how incredible the clinical instructor was at this site. My fingers and toes were crossed.

Incredible doesn't even begin to describe him. Shelley was an amazing combination of knowledge and positivity, while being completely approachable and down to earth. He made each of his students feel important, needed, worthy of teaching and capable of learning. At the time, he had no way of knowing how much that meant to me personally. He had no knowledge as to why I had been transferred to this location. The other students in my clinical group had no idea either. At times it felt like I was playing the game "which one of these things doesn't belong?" That would be me; the nursing student who was thrown out of her last clinical but has to pretend that everything is ok. The one who has nearly constant fear of having to ready a defense, should anyone find out. The one who wonders who might already know. The potential stigma that would follow me through school should this incident become public knowledge was beginning to slowly paralyze me.

Completely overwhelmed, I let feelings of shame and self-doubt creep over me, pushing me deeper and deeper into emotional isolation. I was haunted by the images of my previous instructor's face and couldn't rid my mind of the degrading things she had said about me. I relived those moments over and over again, every day. It felt like madness. It WAS madness that I would allow a single person to have so much power over me. But I had. As my self-esteem nearly bled out, my instructor had different plans for me. Shelley made it impossible for me to check out and give up. Each time I was with him, I felt a powerful connection. Connected to him, to my love of nursing, and the yearning I had at my core to make a difference. He gave to all of us completely and unselfishly, setting example after example of leadership, compassion and dedication. He became my mentor, believing in my potential when I struggled to.

As nursing students, 'potential' is a common theme in our thoughts. What is the potential to pass the next test? What is the potential to master the next skill? And, maybe most importantly, what is the potential of passing our state board exam and finding a job after finishing school? At the time, I didn't realize this new clinical site would drastically increase my potential for securing my first job as a registered nurse. During the weeks that followed, gradually the huge gray cloud over my head began to lift. Degradation turned into determination and my focus returned to making a difference. My self-doubt began to decrease and a feeling of confidence like I had never experienced before replaced it. Shelley spoke about the importance of knowledge and understanding psychiatric process, but also the equal importance of using intuition and the value of the humanity behind the diagnosis. More than ever before, this message spoke to me, inspired me, and empowered me.

During this clinical rotation it became clear to me that the typical Med/Surg job after graduation was not for me. This new world I was experiencing intrigued me. I felt very comfortable in an environment that quite frankly made other students want to never return. Somehow being on a locked admissions unit with 27 very unstable mentally ill patients didn't scare me in the least. In fact, I looked forward to the opportunity to be in this environment. It challenged me in every way possible, and I LOVED it. Then, the most empowering thing imaginable for a nursing student happened. Shelley asked me to consider coming to work for the clinical site after I graduated. For me, it was validation that what I was feeling on the inside was also visible on the outside.

This was the moment when I knew without any doubt I was meant to be a nurse. It felt like I had finally kept my promise to my nine-year-old self. Although her plans were set on being a doctor, I knew in my heart nursing was the right fit for me. Clearly, the car accident that altered my path twenty-three years before was a catalyst. It began my new journey exactly as it needed to be. All that disappointment had only made me more determined. My emotional and physical pain made me even more passionate about helping others who were suffering. With the support of people who loved and believed in me, I had been able to turn tragedy into triumph. Now, I was more than ready to take the next step to realizing my new dream.

After graduation, you prepare for the NCLEX nursing exam, and after that you prepare to find a job. If you're lucky, you pass the exam in one try. If you're really lucky, you have a job offer and position waiting for you upon passing. It appeared that my luck had changed. I passed on the first try, was offered a job, and started as a brand-new baby nurse on day shift. Any new grad will tell you that's like winning the nursing lottery. My head was filled with a mixture of elation and terror. The entire time I was in school my instructors told me time and time again that the first year you actually work as a nurse is when your real learning begins. Basically, nursing school teaches you just enough that hopefully you don't kill somebody during that first year. And so it began, my new mantra, which I pretty much said to myself every day of my first year...I will not kill anybody today, I will not cry today, I will be brave.

Chapter 9

Participation Required

"Optimism is the faith that leads to achievement.
Nothing can be done without hope and confidence."
–Helen Keller

L uckily for me, I had excellent orientation at that first job. Which came in handy on my second day as a brand-new nurse. You see, a nurse didn't show up for her shift, and there wasn't another nurse to cover for her, so I was put in charge of the entire floor. Yep, charge nurse on day two. Welcome to the wonderful world of nursing, where call offs and double shifts are a daily occurrence. Being that it was day two as a new employee and new nurse, there wasn't an opportunity to say no. I just agreed to do it. I said my mantra a lot that day! Once the rest of the team found out I was going to be in charge, Brian, a very brave mental health clinician walked over to me and quietly asked if I had any idea what I was doing. This was the same employee that I had been warned about on day one. I was told he did not cooperate, was not a team player, and generally had a bad attitude. Instead of taking offense to the question, I smiled and confidently told him I knew the basics but would really appreciate it if he would be willing to share his knowledge with me. To my surprise, he agreed to help me. And to my delight, on my second day as a nurse, I didn't kill anybody, I didn't cry, and I was brave.

From that day on, I often asked for Brian's cooperation and participation during our sometimes-difficult days. He always helped me and seemed agreeable to do any task that I presented him with. The person that was described to me on day one just didn't seem to exist. Several months later, on a Saturday morning, which was our Friday, I was brave enough to ask him when I would get to meet his alter ego. He chuckled and then looked a little sad. Brian explained that as a mental health clinician he felt his ideas and input mostly fell on deaf ears. This frustrated him and made him angry and at times he would just check out, so he could get through his day. He told me that I was the first nurse who had ever asked for his help and appreciated his participation in making the daily schedule work. Brian conveyed this made him feel needed and important and actually renewed his commitment to helping people. In that moment, I realized that everyone needs a purpose. And it is in participation that purpose is found.

With that thought in mind, I eagerly accepted the offer to be the charge nurse on Saturdays. When I was in that role, I asked for all team members to participate in every aspect of our day. I didn't make assignments, I asked for volunteers. I wanted everyone on the team to know that we were equals and that my title did not trump theirs. After all, I was the new kid on the block. Most of the clinicians I worked with had bachelor's degrees and more than 10 years of experience in the mental health field. What I came to understand was the modus operandi had always been that the nurse was the queen and the clinicians were her subjects. And, you better be a loyal subject, or your days would quickly be filled with the crappiest tasks available. I thought this was outrageous and an incredibly ignorant waste of these individual's passion and talents. I vowed that at least one day a week these people would be heard, and their skills put to good use to make a difference in the lives of our patients. And oh my, the differences we made!

I began to look forward to working on Saturdays, and I believe my team did as well. I liked being in charge, but I most enjoyed collaborating with my team. Working together on solutions made any challenge seem less daunting. I started noticing that not only were my team members participating more but our patients were, as well. There seemed to be a change taking place in the unit. I watched my coworkers become vested and in turn more dedicated to not giving up on our patients, no matter what the situation. By offering a supportive environment to one another, we could better support our patients. This equated to more meaningful interventions, one on one conversations and less punitive outcomes like placing a patient in isolation, or even worse, using restraints. As we participated together, we felt empowered. It seemed like anything was possible. During this time, I started putting more thought into this process and writing those thoughts down. This mentality became the foundation for the therapeutic group I asked our patients to participate in. My goal was to reconnect these people who had been so disconnected as a result of their diagnosis. This disconnection was further complicated by the stigma that exists in our society surrounding mental illness.

The thing about stigma related to mental illness is that it has many components to it. There is certainly judgment from the outside, but the judgment from the inside is just as prevalent. Stigma inside the inner world of mental illness can be extremely damaging as it comes from one's self, their peers, and sometimes the very clinicians that are supposed to be neutral and helpful. In my opinion, the stigma surrounding mental illness is in fact a form of prejudice. Unfortunately, many healthcare workers, along with the general public, are guilty of this. Seeing this from my peers was quite uncomfortable. However, the self-loathing and feelings of worthlessness that my patients exhibited toward themselves and their peers who were also struggling with these issues was truly devastating. They were in a perpetual state of feeling hopeless.

I will not deny that at times this hopeless situation seemed overwhelming to me too. It would have been much easier to walk away than face this dilemma. I think that is one reason burnout and employee turnover is so high in this field. That was the choice. Leave, which many before me did, or stay and try to make a difference. I decided to stay and to change my mantra. It was simple: I will not give up on these people and I will be brave. Not giving up and being brave was essential if I was to succeed. By the time my patients reached my admissions unit, pretty much everyone in their lives had given up on them. Their trust level was at zero and they anticipated being let down again. They expected me to give up on them. I had to be brave because I was about to embark on a non-clinical approach to a very clinically based issue. There was a diagnosis, medications prescribed to treat the diagnosis, behavior therapy, and a corresponding ICD-9 code used for medical billing. Period. We were not to waiver from this methodology. In fact, to do so, was considered challenging the entire system. I mean who did I think I was anyway? I was a new nurse with six months of mental health experience. It turns out my inexperience became my greatest strength.

Chapter 10

Empower to the People

*"Lord save us all from a hope tree that has
lost the faculty of putting out blossoms."*
–Mark Twain

T he great thing about being the newbie is that many times the stuff other people have negative thoughts about hasn't even hit your radar yet. You're all shiny and new and don't really know what you don't know. Yes, it may be an unrealistic view, but for me, it worked. To be clear, I understood the potential threat and considerable danger when interacting with a new client straight off the street. I always was cautious and did not place myself in danger. I followed my CPI (crisis prevention) training to the letter. I asked for assistance from my co-workers and our

Security Department should I need back up. After all, I had a family to go home to that I loved very much. And, the horror stories about what had happened to the nurses before me sent the message home. Be safe. Don't put yourself in a dangerous situation. Which of course, we all did the moment we clocked in and that door locked behind us.

So, how does one go about empowering people when their most basic freedom has been taken away? Every patient on my unit was locked up. They had either hurt themselves, someone else or a combination of. They were not considered safe to be in society. They had burned every bridge they had by the time we met. I think hitting rock bottom pretty much sums it up. So, imagine when the first person they meet is me, a shiny new nurse, who wants to save the world, smiling from ear to ear. I'm sure some of my patients immediately thought, this is a joke, right? How could anyone be that happy to be here? But the truth is, I was, and I found that a smile could disarm anger and almost immediately connect people. So that's what I did a lot. I smiled. When I was happy, nervous or scared out of my mind, I smiled. And, I was brave.

One of my bravest moments was when I put together my therapeutic group I called "Finding H.O.P.E.". I submitted it to Shelley, who was the Director of Nursing, for approval. Since he had been my clinical instructor I did not want him to think he had made a mistake by hiring me. His approval meant the world to me. He was definitely a mentor and someone whom I respected as a nurse, scholar and advocate for mental health issues. There was no clinical aspect to my group, which all the groups on our unit had. Strike one. There was no sound evidence that what I wanted to teach had any merit. Strike two. It was the product of my experiences with my patients and my intuition that I could help patients feel hopeful while being in what seemed a very hopeless situation. Really? Strike three. So, when Shelley called me to his office, I anticipated him telling me that my heart was in the right place, but he could not possibly approve my group. But, he not only approved my group, he validated the method I wanted to teach. He told me he thought my process had real merit. In fact, he gave me kudos for my approach and blew me completely away when he stated that he felt once proven, this had potential to be a new nursing theory. I was speechless and once again overwhelmed with gratitude toward this man. I thanked him and walked out of his office and remembered part of my mantra. I will not cry. As it turned out, crying was a pivotal part of the therapeutic process to finding hope in many cases, for my patients and for myself.

Once you truly have a connection with another human being, it's nearly impossible not to experience what they are experiencing. This is the reason Human Connection is where I believe hope starts. On our unit, as with all the units at our facility, there was a strict policy about touch. No touching allowed between patients, no touching allowed between clinicians and patients. No hand shake, no holding hands, no hugging. None. This was completely foreign to me both personally and professionally. Yes, I understood that clinically, giving a hug to someone who was hypersexual or actively experiencing hallucinations would be counterproductive and possibly even physically dangerous. Yet, many of our severely depressed patients would have benefited from even a small amount of reassuring touch. Here again, one of the most basic human needs was denied to our patients. I struggled with this every day because I disagreed with this policy. I felt it was an outdated method and did more harm than good. It further isolated these already extremely disconnected patients. I had to find another way to connect.

During that first group, I had three or four patients participate. These particular patients were required to attend a certain number of groups per week. Honestly, I believe most of them came to go through the motions of fulfilling their weekly group quota. For me, that was ok because when I thoroughly bombed this group I wouldn't feel as though I did them a disservice. If nothing else, I helped them meet their quota. The first question I asked was whether they felt hopeful, hopeless or somewhere in between. The answer a male patient quickly shouted was "Are you f*** kidding me? Look at us. We've got to be the most hopeless people on earth". And so it began. We had a place to start. I acknowledged his statement and told them all that I did not have a magic wand, all the answers or tools, but I truly wanted to try to help them. The same gentleman, obviously the leader of the group, looked around and told everyone I seemed "legit" and agreed to participate for today. The rest of the patients acquiesced, and we began our journey.

In the same way our DNA makes us human and connects us, a diagnosis can disconnect us. All too often on my team it was an "Us" against "Them" mentality. "They", being the patients, "Us", being the staff. Truth of the matter is that many of the staff I worked with had a mental illness diagnosis of their own. They just had the benefit of a nametag, key to unlock the door, and support system at home. Period. The irony of that was something I pointed out often during my groups. I would try to strip away any barrier I could. Titles like Doctor and Nurse could be misconstrued as authoritarian, which many of our patients had issues with. We literally had to get down to the most basic level of connection. We were interacting as human beings to human beings, nothing more than our DNA connecting us. No titles, no diagnosis's, no stigmas were present. In that simple moment we found out that we were more alike than different. We had just completed our first step towards empowerment and regaining hopefulness.

During the next few days, every person that had attended my group smiled and made eye contact with me as we passed in the hallway. Of course, to most people smiling and making eye contact is part of everyday life. But for these patients, distrust, fear, paranoia, and sometimes hallucinations, made this basic human exchange nearly impossible. Secretly, I was thrilled! Professionally, I knew it was way too soon to be excited or get my hopes up. The irony of that thought made me laugh out loud. This was way before laughing out loud was a thing. In fact, laughing out loud for no apparent reason where I worked was considered a red flag. So, when I realized what I had just done, I looked around to see who might have heard me. Turns out none of my co-workers were within earshot. Excellent! However, in front of me a patient was coming out of his room. As I walked by, hoping he had not heard me, he inquired, "what's so funny?" On any other day, at any other time, I probably would have said "nothing, never mind" and just kept walking. Except, he had come to my class. I owed him more than that. He had been brave and stayed. He had let his defenses down and allowed himself to be open to a new possibility. I turned, smiled and told him what had made me laugh out loud. He didn't think it was quite as funny as I had, but it started a conversation between us. It was just a normal conversation between two human beings, connecting over nothing important really, just connecting.

Chapter 11

Identity Theft

*"What is true of the individual will be
tomorrow true of the whole nation if individuals
will but refuse to lose heart and hope."*
–Mohandas Gandhi

Consider for a moment your own identity. For most of us, identifying who we are is pretty easy. We are sons and daughters, brothers, sisters, mothers & fathers. We identify with our ethnicity, heritage and culture. Furthermore, we identify with our career path or our life purpose. The idea of identity for most of us is solid. Our identity may change over time with our life experiences, but most of us clearly know who we are through this evolution.

This concept changes dramatically with a mental illness diagnosis. It is as though the person slowly disappears, and the diagnosis takes over. Parents lose their children and children lose their parents. I cannot tell you how heartbreaking it is to listen to a mother sob and beg for her child to be brought back from the hold of schizophrenia. Worse yet, seeing the same mother give up, believing her child is forever lost. She can no longer bear feeling hopeless and helpless. Unfortunately, this was not a singular occurrence. Time and time again, families were divided and destroyed by this situation. The grief a family endures, believing a member of their family is lost to chronic mental illness, is similar to that of actually losing a loved one to death. They are no longer the Jones family, family of four. They are now the Jones family, who has a child with Schizophrenia, divided by the stigma of mental illness, forever mourning the loss of a bright future. Some feel guilty that they should have seen this coming and somehow prevented it. Others are suspicious of which side of the family this disease has come from. Many, on some level, are angry at a system that could not cure their child.

Unless you consider court ordered medications, ECT (electric current therapy) and fifteen-minute safety checks normal, there was nearly nothing I would consider normal in these patient's lives while receiving treatment. We told them when to eat, what they could eat, where they could eat, and with whom they could eat. Why? Because this is the way we kept order and boundaries intact. We control a patient's day to restore order and yet I would argue it creates more disorder. These patients had lost total control of their lives due to mental health issues, sexual abuse, drug abuse, and domestic violence. They came to us broken and hopeless, and most of the time, not by choice. To further exacerbate this, we take all their personal items, deciding which items they may keep and which items they may earn back. Yes, this is in the name of safety, for them and for everyone else on the unit. I do not argue that safety comes first. It does. However, I believe we underestimate the value of these last few personal items that are stripped away at what must be one of the most hopeless moments for them. But we see it as a part of a mandatory process that must take place in order to keep them safe and protect all who are now interacting with them. When a patient has lost their family, their home, their mind, and their dignity, the personal items in that trash bag they are admitted with are sometimes all they have left of their identity. And we take them. Leaving them without a shred of their identity to hold on to.

With each admission, I found myself feeling more lost, overwhelmed, and powerless to help my patients or their families. After only a year, I was already feeling the effects of the emotional rollercoaster ride some of my patients had endured over a lifetime. On the outside I was brave and still tried to smile. Inside, I was starting to fear that I was not making a positive impact on my patients. The realization that these patients came to us with a lifetime of mental illness, and often with case history too horrible to comprehend began to paralyze me. I felt like I was losing my own ability to remain hopeful. Looking back, I can see that not only was my own identity being challenged, but my humanity too. It became a matter of survival. Go to work, do the work, come home from work. Clearly, I was starting to check out, like so many before me. I was losing the very thing I was working so hard to restore.

At some point, the Universe seems to give us what we need. Most of the time, we don't recognize it as anything remotely needed. In fact, sometimes the thing we need is placed in front of us as an extraordinary obstacle. For me, this appeared on my path as a workman's comp injury. During the time I was going to work, doing the work and coming home from the work, I fell at work. I was completing safety checks in an isolation room, a room where no food or drinks were allowed. Somehow this female patient had been able to get a drink into her room. As I walked briskly into her room, doing my work, just focusing on getting the task done, I slipped on whatever it was that she had poured on the floor. My left leg went out from underneath me, I soared into the air, with my weight coming down on my right leg, hitting the rest of the liquid on the floor, and then landing with my right knee bending backwards.

To this day, I can still remember the cracking sound and burning sensation on the front of my knee. Imagine a stalk of celery breaking and then having a hot poker touch your kneecap. That pretty much sums it up. Well, crap, this was not on my radar for today. I was supposed to go to work, do the work and come home. Now I had to deal with this inconvenience. And, I wanted to know who was responsible for letting this patient have something to drink in her room. I got up, mad as h***. Someone was going to answer for this obviously avoidable accident. But the pain in my knee was a little more distracting than I had first anticipated. But, I was tough. This fall was not going to stop me from finishing my work. Not only would it stop me, it would effectively REMOVE me. My own identity and many of the things I identified with were about to be taken away.

Chapter 12

Disguised Blessing

"He, who has health, has hope; and
he who has hope, has everything."
–Thomas Carlyle

I vaguely remembered the protocol we were taught in orientation for reporting an injury. I went to Ruth, my charge nurse, reported what happened, and down played it as much as I could. With all the work she had to do, this was more of a nuisance than anything for her. She too seemed perturbed that this could have been prevented and wanted to find out who had broken safety protocols by allowing this woman to have a drink in her room. For a while, this became the priority. Surprisingly, no one fessed up to the crime. Then the pain in my knee was nearly unbearable. It was becoming apparent that I might have seriously injured myself. I really didn't have time for this crap. So, I finished my shift and conceded that my next stop was to the clinic where I thought I would be instructed to just take it easy for a few days.

By the time I drove myself to the clinic, my knee was throbbing, and I was struggling to hold it together, but I was still mad, which actually helped. When I got out of the car, I gingerly put weight on my leg to stand, and found that I could not. Cussing under my breath and refusing to ask for help, I managed to get out of the car and then hopped across the parking lot into the clinic. Once inside, I continued to hop across the waiting room to check in. Several patients in the waiting room watched me approach, but then went back to reading their magazines. Apparently, I was not the first person they had seen hop into the clinic. The staff also watched, but didn't ask if I needed help, which in my current mood was just fine. I wanted to get in and out, go home and put this day behind me.

Having worked full time for the last twenty-five years, and never having an injury on the job, I was seriously unprepared for what awaited me. The amount of paperwork was daunting and the telling and re-telling of what happened was quite intense. It was as if I was on trial. I was asked to give both verbal and written accounts of the incident, including the time and location, and whether or not there were any witnesses to my fall. When I answered that there was not a witness to my fall, I felt like there was a shift. Was I being paranoid, or did these people suddenly seem a little more skeptical? However, during this time, the pain became overwhelming, and I finally realized that I was seriously injured. Realization suddenly hit me. As a nurse, my job was very physical.

Plus, I worked on a unit where being physically fit kept me safe. If I truly had a significant injury, I most likely would not be able to go back to work.

During the exam, I could no longer hold back my tears. These tears were a mixture of anger, fear and reaction to the excruciating pain I had with even the slightest movement. I felt like I was in some kind of horrible dream. I wanted to wake up or at least turn back the clock. What had seemed like such a mundane task just a few hours ago, was the catalyst in a chain reaction that would change the course of my career entirely. After a thorough assessment, my worst-case scenario was presented to me. The doctor was very concerned that I had a significant injury. She believed it was either a meniscus or ACL tear, or possibly both. Effective immediately, I was non-weight bearing. I received orders for pain meds, crutches, RICE, and an MRI.

Quickly, the fighter in me thought, "let's fix this" and move on. My MRI was scheduled within a day or two. While I waited, I tried to stay positive. I was completely compliant, the picture of what a cooperative patient should look like. I kept telling myself that the MRI would confirm the injury; I would have surgery and move on. I could be back on my team within six weeks. This was going to be no more than a little bump in the road during the beginning of my nursing career. I knew lots of nurses that had injuries and came back, continuing in the profession for many years. Maybe I would have to ice my knee after a long shift, but that was certainly do-able. This was not going to keep me from living out my dream.

When the MRI came back negative, no one was more surprised than I was. The pain in my knee had not really decreased and was only manageable with the pain meds and lots of ice. The doctor who had assessed me also seemed surprised, but quickly changed her direction of care after seeing the MRI results. I was immediately put back on full weight bearing, sent back to work on light duty, was to start PT and "work through the pain". When I explained that I still had very intense pain, I got that same feeling that there was a shift. Somehow, this very caring physician now seemed a little skeptical. Maybe I was just being paranoid. Maybe I wasn't.

Unfortunately, I came to realize that mental illness is not the only area where stigma still exists. It is present BIG TIME in the workman's comp arena. I began to feel like I had a stamp on my forehead. A stamp that said, "her pain can't possibly be this bad and she must be trying to milk the system." When I went to PT it was through the workman's comp doctor. They also seemed to be skeptical about the amount of pain I was still having. Often, they pointed out to me that my MRI was negative, and I needed to realize that the pain wasn't going to go away immediately, and I just needed to work through it. The fact that I was a nurse and felt like I knew my body pretty well didn't seem to matter. The diagnosis was clear. My knee looked normal for a forty something year old female. There was no injury, so get over it already. The continued PT felt like it made my knee worse. When I tried to convey this, I was asked if I really wanted to get better. Here I was, a patient in pain, relying 100% on these professionals to help me get well. Instead, not only was I not being taken seriously, but I was being challenged daily as to whether my pain was actually real. Seriously?

The stigma didn't stop there. I faced a challenge at work too. My injury meant I couldn't work on the floor as a nurse. I could do clerical work, but not true nursing. I was given the option of doing really insignificant tasks like filing, or I could stay at home.

I needed a paycheck, so I agreed to work wherever they assigned me. I understand that this put a strain on my team and I think they assumed I would be back pretty quickly after the negative results on the MRI. So, when I continued to be on light duty I think some of them questioned my motives. Support seemed to turn to suspicion. Why wasn't I coming back? What was wrong with me? Was this all just psychological? The shift I felt was palpable. I no longer felt like part of my team. I felt like an outsider.

Luckily, I had Judy, a nurse manager who was very supportive and didn't think I was "faking it." In fact, it was her kindness and support that led me to get a second opinion. Which for the record, is not an easy task when your entire workman's comp team thinks you're just fine. Plus, there was a negative MRI backing them up. But for the first time, that didn't matter. Judy just listened to me, the person she had hired, not the workman's comp employee that I had become. I remember telling her I felt like I was beginning to lose my mind. I really couldn't believe I still had this much pain, and nothing was wrong. I was feeling worn down by all the skepticism. The truth was, I felt hopeless. I was starting to believe that no matter what I did this situation was not going to get better. I had zero power left.

Chapter 13

Second Chances

"We must accept finite disappointment,
but never lose infinite hope."
–Martin Luther King, Jr.

W hen you feel hopeless and powerless, the best thing you can hope for is a supportive advocate. In my case, mine was a supercharged nurse manager named Judy. She was ready for a fight. There was no way she was going to let these people push me around anymore. She was my champion. And, boy did I need one. Her energy began to restore my energy and my reservoir of hope began to fill. Before I knew it, I had a second opinion lined up with a doctor that I had personal experience with through my son. You see, when your kid breaks a lot of bones you get to know orthopedic docs. As fate would have it, the doctor that helped with my son's wrist happened to specialize in knees AND he was on the approved workman's comp doctor list. The sun was starting to shine again.

During my first visit, I mentioned to Dr. K that we had met before. He looked a little puzzled, trying to remember my face. I told him it had been awhile since we had seen each other. I explained that he had helped my son with his fractured wrist, who was the kid that played guitar, with the big hair. His face lit up immediately and he smiled, he remembered him. The conversation quickly turned to my son, his wrist, and his music. In that moment, I was no longer a patient, just a proud Mom. It felt so good to talk about something other than my problems. I felt completely carefree. The conversation eventually turned back to me, but it seemed so different than previous conversations I had about my knee. This time, I told my story and really felt like my doctor was listening to me. There was no judgment, just fact-finding questions and responses.

The first thing I learned was that MRIs are only 87% accurate. That meant there was a 13% chance something was missed. It was unlikely, but possible nonetheless. He wanted to start treatment by doing a series of injections in my knee. Sometimes knees that are injured and heal remain painful. I wasn't thrilled by the idea of having injections in my knee but at least it was an attempt to help me eliminate the pain. The first injection was into the side of my knee joint and honestly wasn't that bad. However, the pain that followed the next few days was excruciating. I was told this was normal and would dissipate in a few days. The pain from the injection did ease up, but the original pain remained unchanged.

My doctor was not discouraged and explained that sometimes the first injection wasn't enough and that's why a series of injections are needed. This time he placed the injection into the front of my knee, which nearly sent me off the table. He actually said this was good because the cortisone was placed in the area with the most inflammation. I trusted this doctor and hoped that my knee pain would disappear this time and I could get on with my life.

When I had requested a change in doctors, I also asked to be seen by a different physical therapist. I chose Marne, a very caring and gentle physical therapist that had helped both my husband and I recover from previous neck and back injuries. I didn't realize just how much this decision would impact the course of my treatment. Once again, my connection with another human being would have a dramatic effect on my life. Since the initial injury to my knee, I would hear a popping noise that intermittently produced pain. It seemed that the more physical therapy I did, the more the popping and corresponding pain increased. I had reported this several times to my previous physical therapist and was basically ignored. However, when Marne heard my knee pop during one of our sessions, she became quite alarmed. In fact, she told me that she would not do any more PT with me because it could be making my knee worse. This is exactly what I had been thinking all along, but those thoughts had been unheard until now. Marne put a call into Dr. K with her thoughts and before I knew it, I was scheduled for exploratory surgery.

Talk about a rollercoaster ride, which in the literal sense of the word I love. But this ride had been full of anything but love. The last few months of my life had felt like an endless road of disbelief and isolation. I was an empty shell of the bright and shiny new nurse I had been only a few months ago. I had been beaten down by the very system that is there to help people when they are injured on the job. The initial clinicians assigned to evaluate and help me had done nothing but hinder my recovery. The worst part was that all of this was based on one negative test result. The clinical data outweighed the symptoms being reported by the human being in front of them. And then it hit me. The parallel between what I was experiencing and what my patients experienced was undeniable. They faced the judgment of a clinical diagnosis that often deprived them of their humanity every day. I decided right then and there to use this experience to better serve others.

Honestly, I don't remember all the details of the day of my surgery. But I can still see the kindness in Dr. K's eyes, as he reassured my husband and I before they took me back to do the surgery. He was confident they would figure out what was wrong with my knee and fix it. My internal dialogue was absolutely the opposite. I had been told for so long that there was nothing wrong with my knee. What if I woke up and was told they found nothing? Because just like the MRI showed, there was NOTHING wrong with my knee. I was nearly in a state of panic thinking about how I would face this scenario, having to explain that I really did feel pain in my knee even though they found NOTHING. What would my family think? Would they continue to support me? I already knew what my coworkers thought. I couldn't deal with the thought of returning to work after the surgery found NOTHING and knowing they all thought I was either crazy or trying to milk the system. How had I gotten to such a place of NOTHING?

When I started to wake up from surgery, I could vaguely make out the conversation my husband and Dr. K were having. I heard them talking about a "flap". Turns out, Dr. K had found a large tear in my meniscus, a tear that the MRI had missed. I wasn't crazy after all. There really had been SOMETHING causing the pain in my knee. Hallelujah! I was groggy but so incredibly grateful to finally have an explanation for the pain that had burdened both my mind and my body for way too long. However, I instantly felt anger, as well. Actually, it was more like rage, pointed directly toward all those people who had prolonged my suffering because they refused to listen to me. I wanted each and every one of them to know how much they had failed me so that they would never again fail another human being. I wanted to be vindicated. I wanted to scream, "I told you so". I wanted to rub their mistake in each of their faces. Obviously, I was in a very dark place, quite possibly, the world's biggest victim.

Chapter 14

People not Patients

"There is no medicine like hope, no incentive so great, and no tonic so powerful as expectation of something tomorrow."
–Orison Swett Marden

I mmediately after surgery, I was able to put my full weight on my leg and walk to the bathroom. It was truly amazing, just having surgery and feeling no pain! ZERO. I could not believe it at first. I anticipated the pain that I had come to expect with every step, but it was non-existent. I quickly came to the realization that I had two choices. I could wallow in self-pity for all the suffering I had needlessly endured and remain a victim or, I could trade in my anger for acceptance and choose to be a survivor. I chose to be a survivor and use this experience, with all its pain and hopelessness, to help others in the future. First, I needed to thank the people who had helped me. I wanted each of them to understand how truly grateful I was for their support, encouragement and belief in me. Without it, I don't think I would have made it through this ordeal. Each ONE of them had played a role in my life; further proving to me that ONE human being really can make a difference in another human being's life.

During my conversations of gratitude, I found a common thread. Although I was giving tremendous credit to each of these individuals for helping me, in fact saving me, they all received the message nearly the same way. It was as though they felt their part had been very small. They were just doing their jobs and it was no big deal. These people had ultimately turned the tide of my entire story and yet they truly felt they had not really done all that much. They didn't see themselves as the heroes that I saw them as. Don't get me wrong; they were all accepting of my appreciation. But they felt what they had done for me was routine and part of what they did each day in their professional roles. What I felt was heroics, was simply ho hum to them. I had been saved by these people, but they felt like they were simply doing their jobs. How could they not see the profound affect they had on my life? Instead, each of them reflected back to me how grateful THEY were to be a part of my healing process. My being whole again was all the thanks they needed, and I believed this to be true for every single one of them.

The complete opposite was true for the medical professionals I reached out to that had not supported me. I suppose my approach with them was certainly less than grateful. In my defense, I did wait until my anger subsided and only wanted to notify them, so they could do better with future patients; an educational interaction, that's it. What I received was a mix of responses. First, I concluded rather quickly that neither my knee nor I were memorable. Maybe it was because I no longer limped with a cane. Or maybe it was because I no longer resembled the beaten down victim they had seen so many times.

Some of the people I'd seen three times a week literally looked at me as though they had never met me. When I tried to explain the situation and how it had been resolved, I didn't get a positive response from any, except for one person. It was the receptionist at the Physical Therapy office that had showed me empathy from the very beginning. She remarked how sorry she was that I had gone through all of this and was so happy that I was better. The rest of the people I spoke to said very little. I suppose they may have been fearful about what my intentions were.

What I took away from this experience was that all these people were medical professionals whose job it was to help their patient. They were all working with the same collective clinical data, the same history and physical information, the same MRI results. The only difference was that some of them had no prior experience with the patient and some of them knew this patient on a personal level. Could that factor alone really have made all the difference in the outcomes? I believe that all the medical professionals involved in my case provided the care they felt was warranted, based on the clinical data available to them. I also believe that Marne and Dr. K went above and beyond the basic understanding of that clinical data based on a personal connection with their patient. They were compelled to help the human being in front of them because they actually SAW the human being in front of them.

From that realization came my conviction to do the same. I would be a better nurse to all my patients. I would see the PERSON in front of me, not just a patient. I would continue to use the clinical data as part of my assessment, but no longer would it be the majority of what I saw. I wanted to do better. I knew I could do better because someone had done better for me, and as a result, I was in the position to be able to pay it forward. By seeing the human being in front of me, I knew I would be more invested and unwilling to give up. This fundamental change in thinking allowed me to better connect with the people I was trying to help. Instead of being apprehensive because of clinical data or case history, I was able to gain trust and develop a rapport much quicker. In turn, this enabled therapeutic conversations to begin almost immediately. It was through these conversations that true healing began.

For the next several months, I continued my work at the Fort. I felt empowered and wanted to empower those around me, both clinicians and clients alike. Each day, I went to work determined to make a difference. And for a while I did. I was even offered a promotion to Nurse II, the coveted charge nurse position. I was thrilled! However, this position would not be on my current team. That excited me even more. I could take what I had learned and use it to help another team, especially in my new leadership role. Life was good. I could see myself staying at the Fort and helping people struggling with mental health issues indefinitely. I had found my career path as a nurse in less than two years from graduating. Most of my peers were still figuring out what they wanted to do. Many of them were stuck in Med/Surg at a hospital just doing their time until something else became available. But not me! I was working my dream job. Two weeks before I transferred to my new position, I received a phone call that changed everything.

Chapter 15

Alabama

"Keep all special thoughts and memories for lifetimes to come. Share these keepsakes with others to inspire hope and build from the past, which can bridge to the future."
–Mattie Stepanek

T he leap of faith I was about to take could be considered ludicrous, unless you considered WHOM I had faith in. Once again, Shelley would be responsible for changing the course of my nursing career. He wanted me to consider going to work as an Assistant Director of Nursing with his partner, Wade. At first, I thought he had to be kidding. I had just accepted a full-time charge nurse position at the Fort. I couldn't possibly back out now. But the story he told me was too compelling not to consider. A large skilled nursing facility had pretty much cleaned house with their nursing management team. Wade had accepted the position as ADON over the long-term care area but they needed a second ADON to manage the Alzheimer's and Rehab units. They had also hired a new Director of Nursing who he could not say enough good things about. Turns out, she was even better than he said she was.

Before I met her though, I would need to interview with the Executive Director, Roslyn. I was given the impression that this interview was simply a matter of following the facility's hiring protocol. My recommendation from Wade had sealed the deal since she pretty much adored him. Maybe it was my intuition at work, maybe my self-doubt, but man was I nervous. I had interviewed many times before for much higher-level positions without feeling this way. Perhaps it was guilt about my potential sudden departure from the passionate work I had just begun. Work I was leaving for nothing more than the dangled carrot of a significant pay increase. No matter the reason, the uneasiness that existed deep within me that day usually only presented itself in threatening situations. It was almost as if my fight or flight response engaged as I walked into her office. My mind was racing as I stepped forward to greet her, with my best impersonation of a sincere smile, while I silenced my thoughts to turn around and run. This feeling would return again and again over the next eighteen months.

As it turned out, those thoughts seemed to be unfounded because the interview went really well. Wade was there to help guide the interview and his presence was reassuring. He and Roslyn exchanged glances often and seemed very comfortable with one another. The easy conversation between them allowed me to let my guard down a bit. To be clear, this person had been responsible for firing the entire previous nursing team. I viewed her as someone who was at the very least to be respected, if not feared. However, the thing that relaxed me the most during our time together was her incredible belly laugh. When I sat down at a small table in her office, I leaned on the table a little too much and it nearly toppled over. I was mortified at my clumsiness, but she found it to be quite funny. I don't remember exactly what she said, but it was a mixture of sarcasm and humor, both traits that I greatly enjoy in others. I left that interview admiring her strength to make necessary changes but also liking the fun-loving side of her who could laugh. I really wanted to be part of her team. There was just one more thing left to do before that could happen.

The first time I spoke to Abigail, her heart spoke to mine. She was originally from Alabama and had a very thick southern accent, along with a relaxing cadence that immediately soothed me. Our first conversation was supposed to be an interview, but it felt more like two friends talking. I suppose the fact that we both had come from psychiatric nursing backgrounds gave us something to talk about and yet our connection was so much more than that. My nursing experience seemed to matter much less to her than my people skills did. It was as if she was trying to figure out what kind of human being I was. The longer we spoke, the more I felt like we were kindred spirits. It was like we were long lost friends reconnecting, instead of complete strangers talking for the first time. It never felt like an interview, and when we hung up, I knew the job was mine.

Over the next eighteen months, the job proved to be nothing like what I had anticipated, and it challenged me in every way possible. Honestly, I don't know what I would have done without Abigail during this time. Yes, her professional role was my supervisor, but she became much more than that. She was my mentor, my sounding board, my confidant, my teacher, my protector, and my friend. Abigail had a profound way about her that impacted people in the most delightful way. I loved to watch her interact with our residents and their families. As soon as she began to speak her relaxing cadence was like a spell cast out, spreading warmth and reassurance. Some people might call it Southern charm, but it was more powerful than that. Her inner light was so bright, and she had a carefree way about her that was disarming. You just couldn't say no to her.

Abigail always knew what battles to choose. She was a warrior and a ferocious advocate for patient rights. She also fought hard for her staff. No matter what we had to face, it was always reassuring to know that she was by our side facing it with us. She could enter a volatile situation, diffuse it and come out on the other side seemingly unscathed. Except, the longer I knew her, the more I understood that there was a toll taken, a burden that she alone accepted without concern. When someone is so dedicated to helping others, and they do it so well and with such ease, it's easy to forget that they too might need support. Abigail was one of those people. She gave and gave without ever asking for anything in return. Her ability to love and accept people even when they've wronged her was astounding. She represented the truest form of unconditional love and wisdom.

I am uncertain whether she was born with these gifts or if they were instilled to her during her childhood. Her loving relationship with her parents and family was very apparent. Maybe it was a bit of both. The stories of her childhood were a magical blend of love, life lessons and a bit of mischief. I could listen to her reminisce about her childhood adventures for hours. She would start to tell a relatively benign story and then suddenly it would take a wild turn and become a tall tale. I absolutely loved it when she would pause, and with a twinkle in her eye, say "there's always a story". At that point, I knew I was in store for a delightful accounting of an event in her life. No matter what the subject was, her stories had a way of touching you and making you feel connected to her life and even more connected to your own. Once again, the power of human connection was at play in my life.

To this day, Abigail is still one of the best listeners I know. No matter what the subject is, it matters to her. That alone has a way of making someone feel special. It also has a certain power to promote hope. I believe that when a person truly feels that they are being heard, it is cathartic. It allows true feelings to be spoken without fear. That is an extremely powerful gift to bestow. Abigail often shared this this priceless gift with me, allowing me to release negative thoughts and replace them with empowered ones. She also had the ability to share her wisdom clearly after listening with intent. Something that will always stay with me that she said was: "you've gotta love 'em, but you know them". Which to me meant, love unconditionally, but also understand whom you love. Loving an alcoholic unconditionally won't make them stop drinking, but that doesn't make the love you have for them mean any less. In that wisdom, so simply put, lives complete freedom.

Chapter 16

Losing Marbles

"Hope is the thing with feathers, that perches in the soul
And sings the tune without the words, and never stops at all."
–Emily Dickinson

After working for a large health care company in corporate America, I quickly figured out that I might be a better fit in a smaller environment. When I saw a job post for an admissions nurse at Hospice of St. John's, a non-profit hospice company, my heart soared. This might be a place where I could do really good work. Plus, I always had this "weird" feeling when one of my patients died. I didn't know then that the "weird" feeling wasn't really weird at all. It's called being comfortable around death. And, many people consider it as having a "heart for hospice".

I think I always knew deep inside that I looked at death a little differently than most people. Turns out there were other people who felt exactly the same way. I was about to discover once again that I could feel passionate about nursing.

Having true passion for helping people is definitely required for working in hospice. It's that passion that carries you during the demands and helps one to continuously refuel. This is especially necessary when you're an admissions nurse. Each new family you meet with is depending on you to help them understand the road that lies ahead. In many cases, a terminal prognosis has been given to them only hours before you arrive. The shock of a life ending diagnosis for himself or herself or a dearly loved family member is written all over their faces. And then there are the pre-existing family dynamics that further complicate an already complicated situation. The person who is choosing hospice may be making this choice for someone who can no longer choose for him or herself. Or, the person who needs hospice may be making this decision against the wishes of their family. No matter what the situation may be, as an admissions nurse, you must be resilient and able to meet each family's unique challenges.

For me, I felt like I could meet any challenge if I focused on establishing a human connection first, rather than focusing on the hospice admission. This certainly wasn't an easy task most of the time. But, I hadn't chosen to be a hospice admission nurse because it was easy. I chose this line of work because I truly wanted to make an impact on people's lives when they were most vulnerable. I felt like I could be a champion in their greatest time of need. Most families need someone to lead them through the unthinkable task ahead and reassure them that not only can this process be therapeutic, but also that hospice focuses on life, not death. In fact, when the "sic" is taken out of hospice what remains is hope, both figuratively and literally. This is where my mission began with each person or family I met with. Connect with them on a basic human level, earn their trust, be their champion, and return hope to their lives. In theory, it is a noble endeavor. However, in reality, no matter how valiant the effort, the outcome is a far cry from success. Unless of course, you redefine the definition of success. Then everything changes.

Over the next eighteen months, there were many ups and some significant downs. I began to realize some families were so disconnected, it was nearly impossible to establish any connection with them. During these meetings, I was so grateful for my psychiatric nursing background. It helped me set boundaries during frantic and often chaotic arguments between family members. I quite literally had to establish the rules of engagement; no yelling or name-calling and only one person may speak at a time. And although some of these families ended up not admitting to hospice, at least a respectful dialogue had begun, and a seed had been planted. This was the new way I began to define my success. Yes, an admission was still my goal, because that was what my employer expected, but on a personal level it became more than that. I wanted to plant the seed of hope, one family at a time.

At the risk of sounding arrogant, I could not be stopped. No matter what the scenario would be, I would finalize the admission. More than one hospice company would often meet with the family and they would still choose Hospice of St. John. I'd be sent out to do what we called an "informational" and next thing you know, they were admitting to us. This pattern continued over and over again. Rarely did I meet with a family and was told they were not ready to admit. It felt wonderful to be helping all these people. I did receive kudos for my abilities, but I believe it wasn't me who was succeeding. I know without a doubt, my method was the true success story. Once I established a human connection, the rest came so easily. By building trust on a very basic human level, families were more open to share their feelings. After that, they welcomed the ability to participate in what the rest of their life was going to look like. Which then led them to a place of empowerment and ultimately hope.

I too felt empowered and hopeful. I could not wait to meet my next family. There was no greater joy for me than to begin my day knowing that I might be able to deliver a message of hope to people in their greatest time of need. And for a time, it was simply magical. Until the day it all ended quite abruptly. I knew Hospice of St. John was struggling financially. I knew there had been two waves of layoffs, but I had survived. I can still remember it as if it was said to me yesterday, "don't worry, your job is safe, they will always need an admissions nurse." Within days of those words being spoken, I was called into HR and told I was being laid off. I was assured that this decision was not based on my productivity and that I had done nothing wrong. They simply could not afford to pay me. They also made sure I knew I could collect unemployment. But I really didn't care about that. All I wanted was to know that somehow the message of hope would continue to be planted. I asked how they were going to admit new patients without an admission nurse. The looks on their faces said it all. Approximately six months later, the doors to Hospice of St. John closed for the final time.

I'm a big believer that when one door closes another opens. Sometimes when said door slams shut, it's harder to walk through the next one. But I was on a mission of hope, so I had to be brave. I had no interest in collecting unemployment. I needed to find another position where I could continue to speak my message. Then I remembered an email I had received just hours before I was laid off. It was from a recruiter of a large hospice and home health company that was looking for a clinical liaison for their hospice team. Within 24 hours I applied and just a few days later I was talking to the regional sales manager, Jennifer. She was dynamic and exuded positivity. I immediately felt a connection with her. We talked about my ability to impact the community on a much larger level because of this company's powerful presence in the market. I wanted nothing more than to be part of Jennifer's team. So, I jumped through that door.

For the next few months this new position was everything Jennifer said it would be. Her team was indeed dynamic, and it felt like we could accomplish anything. She was inspirational when she spoke to the team, building confidence in us to be the best. For a time, it seemed as though we were the best. Our census climbed to an all-time high. We captured clients in areas of the market that previously seemed unattainable. We were on fire. And then the unthinkable happened. Jennifer announced that she was leaving the company. As she said the words I fought back tears. I looked around the room and many of my peers showed the same emotion. We were all devastated. For me personally, I realized Jennifer was the true reason I had gone to work for this company. My connection with her had given me hope that there was something better ahead for me. She had given me the opportunity to share what I cared about so deeply and then demanded that I be an active participant in that belief. She was exactly what I needed at that time in my life.

What I didn't need, was to be involved in what was coming. I think I would best describe it as chaos. Without Jennifer, our team began to crack. People started to leave and new people with new agendas started to enter. The company's brand became more important than the mission to help people. I just could not drink that Kool-Aid. I felt completely lost and hopeless. How could something that had seemed so promising end like this? Within months of me leaving, the company was swallowed up by another organization. Had I stayed, I would have faced another lay off as some of my team members did. As another door closed, I started to question a lot of things in my life. Probably the most significant question was whether I could ever be happy working for someone else again.

Chapter 17

3:22

"You are not here merely to make a living. You are here in order to enable the world to live more amply, with greater vision, with a finer spirit of hope and achievement. You are here to enrich the world, and you impoverish yourself if you forget the errand."
–Woodrow Wilson

As the last door was closing, I thought I was feeling "off" because of the stress. I literally felt like it was all I could do to get out of bed and show up for work, let alone be the energetic person they expected me to be. In addition to finding out I basically had zero hormones left, it turned out I was about to be diagnosed with a fairly significant health issue. After seeing my regular doctor, I was sent to an endocrinologist. Apparently, my thyroid was not functioning, and I had developed a nodule on my thyroid. After an ultrasound, my doctor suggested we treat my hypothyroidism with medication and watch the nodule. It was during this time I started having trouble sleeping. No matter what time I went to bed, I would wake up in the early morning. The strangest thing was the time I woke up. When I looked at the clock, it was almost always 3:22 am.

As a clinical liaison, I had the opportunity to establish connections in the community via marketing events and other community activities. On one occasion I was invited to a charity event where a mutual friend introduced me to a very interesting woman. She was bubbly and extremely friendly, and we hit it off right away. After the event ended, we exchanged contact information and promised to keep in touch. Over the next few months we often met for coffee or lunch. She told me about her future goals to grow her home care business and branch out to the assisted living arena. I was intrigued by her charisma and ability to interact with people so easily. I also liked the fact that she made her own hours as a business owner. Her life seemed perfect to me. When she asked me to join her as she took her business to the next level, I immediately agreed. The pace was much slower than my previous position and as I continued to deal with health issues, this new opportunity seemed perfect.

For a time, our partnership felt perfect. I enjoyed a honeymoon period free from quotas and agendas, but I had no clue how quickly my life was about to turn upside down once more. The charismatic woman I had met just months before was disappearing before my very eyes. The relaxed conversations we once shared now became heated debates over the simplest things. Walking on eggshells whenever we were together was my new normal, I never knew what was going to upset her. Caregivers reported that she was yelling and speaking disrespectfully to them. The entire direction of our path was changing, and I found out there would be no assisted living. I knew I had made a huge mistake. Before I could figure a way out of this, I found myself falling down yet another rabbit hole. She invited me to lunch one last time, only to tell me she had decided not to work with me anymore. I was shocked. My insomnia magnified, and I dreaded going to sleep. I didn't want to face a new reality at 3:22 nearly every morning.

This new reality included me being unemployed, as well as my husband. Todd had lost his job just three weeks before. So here we were. We had no employment, no health insurance and a bank account that was nearly empty. We both felt like we were pretty darn close to rock bottom. I quickly reverted back to my old mantra of "I will be brave and I will not cry." After being completely devastated on July 1st, when I was basically fired, anger I had never felt before rose up in me. That anger turned into a fire that would not be extinguished by anyone or anything. This situation would not break me. I would not only survive this but use it to fuel me. On July 4th, I signed into the State of Colorado website and formed my business, HeartFelts Assisted Living, LLC. While America was celebrating its independence, I was celebrating the beginning of my own.

My husband and I both agreed that leaving Corporate America was the best thing we could do for our family and our future. As a result, Todd also made a huge change in his life. He went back to school and became a Certified Nursing Assistant. As a

CNA, he could help me run our assisted living. We would do this together and together anything was possible. To get us through this transition period, we both cashed out our retirement accounts. That decision took quite a bit of courage because it was our final safety net. If this didn't work out, we quite literally had exhausted our options. We even ran the risk of losing our home. We also had another matter on our minds. Our son was preparing to go to college within the next 12 months. We needed this to work because there was absolutely no way we were putting his dreams of going to college on hold.

During this time, I had a recurring dream from my childhood. There is a tornado coming and I need to get all the people and animals I love into the house so they're safe. Just when I think I have completed this task I realize that someone is missing. The feeling of panic and fear at that moment is so real. I must choose whether to stay safely inside or go out and face the tornado. In the dream, I have always chosen to face the tornado. And now, I face the tornado nearly every night. Sometimes there are multiple tornados. And sometimes it feels like the people I love are purposefully leaving the safety I have created for them. Other times, I have to choose whom I will save because I cannot possibly save everyone. For the first time in months, I am relieved when I wake up, even though I see that once again it is 3:22am.

I am also relieved to have an amazing woman and mentor in my life at this time. Gina and I met when I was a hospice clinical liaison. Gina owned two Assisted Living Homes and was very loyal to a local hospice company for many years. When she agreed to meet with me I was elated. I knew my company might never be her first choice for hospice, but I was hoping we could be her second. The moment we met, I felt a surge of energy and literally felt butterflies in my stomach. My typical introduction meeting lasted 15-20 minutes. Our first meeting lasted nearly two hours. We talked about all sorts of things, but the most important was how we felt about taking care of people. For both of us, caring for people and making a difference in their lives was what truly filled our cups. We also believed that our geriatric population deserved to be treated with the utmost dignity, respect and unconditional love. Gina really understood how hospice could be a significant part of helping her residents age in place and pass peacefully. And, she believed in giving her residents choice. I loved that about her; she understood the importance of choice.

When it came to the separation from my previous business partner, Gina also understood the importance of being honest with me. She recognized something was off and as my friend, she warned me a few weeks before I was blind-sided. So, it was no surprise when I started down this new path to having my own business that she was supportive. In fact, we collaborated through her Home Care Company to admit my first resident. It was a very complicated case that required more care than her team could manage. During this time, I also became an RN consultant for her and her residents. I respected Gina very much for the way she ran her business and how she cared deeply for her residents and staff. She helped me understand that it was possible to care for people on my own terms, and that I didn't need a large corporation to be successful. Simply put, Gina inspired me. When she later asked me to be her business partner and open a third home with her, my aspirations were forever changed.

This clearly was the opportunity of a lifetime. I would have the honor of working alongside this incredibly successful woman. The impact we could make as a like-minded team was endless, certainly more than I could make on my own. And, she was offering me the ability to earn ownership in the house we would open together. The dreams that had been crushed just a few months before would now become a reality. I cannot fully express the joy she brought to my life. Her confidence in me helped restore my belief in myself. In fact, when I look back at our relationship I am still amazed. It began with a human connection that gave me the opportunity to voice my feelings, which lead to Gina asking me to participate in a new path, then ultimately lead me to empowerment and hope.

There's only one thing that's possibly more fantastic about our story. A few months after we began working together full time, the topic of birthdays came up. I shared that I was born in March and Gina said that she and her husband Jim were also born in March. I thought it was kind of cool that we were all Pisces and told her so. But she corrected me and told me that Jim was a Pisces, but SHE was an Aries. At first, I didn't get it. She was born in March, so she should be a Pisces. However, her birthday did not fall between February 19th and March 20th. Her birthday was on March 22nd. I wasn't sure she would believe me, but I told her about waking up at 3:22am for nearly the last year. Once I talked to her about it, I realized something else. Shortly after I met Gina, I stopped waking up at 3:22am. For me, this was confirmation that the Universe had been sending me a message. Finally, I was on the path that had always been meant for me.

Chapter 18

Fostering Hope

> *"Forgiving does not erase the bitter past. A healed memory*
> *is not a deleted memory. Instead, forgiving what we cannot*
> *forget creates a new way to remember. We change the*
> *memory of our past into a hope for our future."*
> **–Lewis B. Smedes**

Before I physically met Janet, I guess you could say her story preceded her. This is pretty common when you are going to provide care for someone. However, her story was anything but expected. As a caregiver, you expect to hear a general health history, what your client likes and dislikes, an overall background. With Janet, nearly every person I spoke to started his or her report with "Where do I begin?" And then it would begin.

I seriously had never heard as many adjectives used to describe an 80-year-old woman before. To repeat these here would only reopen wounds that were very deep at the time. You see, I'm one of those nurses who does not like hearing people labeled like this. In fact, I tend to pretty much ignore most of this part of report. I always want to meet a new client with an open mind.

As I knocked on her door and walked into a very dark room, my mind was open, but I was also taking in everything I saw. Beautiful furniture and paintings furnished the tiny apartment. They were clearly remnants of a life that had once been well lived. In addition to this, was random clutter. There was a half-cup of coffee here and a plate with uneaten food. An unopened newspaper laid on the coffee table alongside the activity schedule, neither of which had been touched. The apartment almost looked abandoned. What I didn't realize then was how much these surroundings reflected the current mental state of the person who lived here. For many reasons, Janet had decided to abandon her once beautifully full life. My learning curve began the moment I walked into her bedroom and attempted to introduce myself.

There had been no response to my knock on the door. There was also no response when I walked into her bedroom and quietly said her name. There was no response when I attempted to introduce myself. For a brief moment, the stillness in the room caused me alarm. Then I saw the rise and fall of her chest. I said her name again and introduced myself again. Very quietly she said, "I don't want to get up". I explained that she didn't have to get up, that I was here whenever she wanted to get up or if she needed anything. She said "ok". As I walked past all the things I had seen on the way in, a feeling of sadness overwhelmed me. How was it possible that this woman, whom had once been a vibrant part of her community, be so very disconnected? What events had led to this broken life? More importantly, how was I going to help her repair it? When I closed her door and sat down just outside her room, my mind, my heart and my soul were flooded with an overwhelming amount of despair.

As I tried to make sense of what I had just seen, I realized that giving up was not an option and my despair transformed into determination. I resolved to help this woman. If I gave up, like so many people had before me, she would also continue to give up and be in this disconnected state for the rest of her life. She wouldn't have to face her demons. Janet would remain paralyzed in the bed that beckoned for her to stay. She would simply continue to fade away from the woman she had once been. Honestly, I think Janet was counting on this. It would be far easier for her to let go of her life than to fight to get it back. The despair I felt after only getting a glimpse of Janet's life had hit me so hard. I could not fathom the intensity of despair she must be living with and how alone and isolated she must feel. I knew I had to find a way to connect with her as a human being if there was to be any chance of helping her. That next step was bigger than I could have ever imagined. Thankfully, I would soon meet an unexpected ally who was not only willing to help, but actually held the key to this closed door.

A short time after I met Janet, I met Kim, her daughter. I knew who she was before she even introduced herself because of her striking resemblance to her mother. Our first meeting was a little intense because of the circumstances. Kim was picking Janet up to take her to an appointment for ECT, electroconvulsive therapy. Obviously, this was not a typical way that a mother and daughter might spend an afternoon together. It was very evident that Kim was struggling with this task. I didn't blame her for having mixed feelings about this treatment. ECT is a fairly extreme procedure, saved for those people who have major depression and do not respond to medication and or psychotherapy. This gave me yet another insight to the depth of despair Janet was experiencing in her life. And, as a daughter myself, it wasn't hard for me to imagine how stressful this must be for Kim. It didn't take long for Kim and I to connect and build trust in one another as daughters and ultimately as allies in the battle to save Janet.

Saving someone who doesn't necessarily want to be saved takes a huge amount of energy and patience. Kim had already been fighting this battle for many years when I met her. She had reached out to her mother's medical doctor who prescribed an antidepressant and medication for Janet's anxiety. When that didn't help, Kim had Janet work with a psychologist. During this time, Kim also tried moving her mother out of her home where she had been very isolated. Janet had lived in multiple communities only to have the same result. She was unhappy and ended up moving back to her large, empty home. The time and energy Kim had spent trying to help her mother find happiness again was staggering. It seemed like the more Kim tried the more Janet retreated into a deeper darker place. After years of this futility, Janet sank so low that she was placed in a geriatric psychiatric unit at a local hospital. This had led to more medications that now included antipsychotics and ultimately ECT. Which by the way, would be court ordered if Janet were not compliant with attending this treatment.

At the root of all this chaos was extreme grief. Norman, the patriarch of their family had died from cancer many years ago. He had been Janet's rock. I believe his death was the catalyst for the unraveling of Janet's life. Norman's death was also felt very deeply by his daughter Kim. But even as she was grieving, Kim took over being the rock for her mother, which further complicated their relationship. Janet demanded more and more of Kim's time, and their relationship became that much unhealthier. Kim often had to choose between taking care of her own two young children and husband or her mother. Which then led to resentment between everyone involved. All families have dynamics, but this family's dynamics were heightened by the death of Norman. He had been the glue that held everything together. Without Norman, his family began to crack and ultimately fall apart, dragging all the members down with it. For me, this reinforced the idea of the true power of human connection. Have it and have everything. Lose it and all can be lost.

In my heart of hearts, I truly believed Janet was lost. Kim had done her very best to be the champion Janet needed. But despite all of Kim's efforts, Janet simply could not move forward passed her grief. The anguish for both mother and daughter was tremendous and it seemed to grow with every interaction they had. At the time, I felt like their connection was actually hurting them. I was honest with Kim about these feelings and thankfully she trusted me enough to hear me out. I gave her my word that I could help her mother, but to do so, I would need to oversee all aspects of her future care. My first step would be to get Janet back home with one on one 24/7 care and a structured daily routine for her. I would enlist a team of dedicated caregivers, a new physician and a counselor to address her depression, ECT and all the medications she was taking. It would have been so easy for Kim to say no, but instead she said yes. Imagine the bravery it took for her to hand over the reins of her mother's care to someone she barely knew. Kim's courage was the catalyst that began a new path for both.

The path ahead was definitely not straightforward and felt more like a series of crossroads. Our first step was getting Janet home with 24/7 home care. When she had gone home previously, she was alone and able to completely shut down. This time, there would be full-time care to make sure that didn't happen. Once she was home we focused on a shift from total isolation to isolating small steps that would take Janet back to wellness. In order to stay home, which is what Janet said she wanted most, she would need to be compliant with this new structured daily routine. We started with simply coming to the kitchen to eat her meals. Then we worked on taking a shower, getting dressed and staying up for small periods of time before retreating to her bedroom. During this time, we also addressed the numerous medications Janet was taking and her ECT treatments. A large majority of her medications were sedating her and the ECT was significantly impacting her memory. Under the guidance of her current PCP and the addition of a new wellness doctor, we were able to gradually discontinue most of her medications and end the ECT treatment. Simultaneously we began intensive weekly counseling to address Janet's grief and depression.

After several months of being in her home, we all came to the realization that Janet would never be able to truly move forward while surrounded by everything that reminded her of a life she had once lived but lost so abruptly. The pull of the past was stronger than the hope of a new future. My next step for Janet required another leap of faith from Kim. I felt compelled to not give up on Janet and believed that we could help her the most in a homelike environment. The home I wanted to bring her to was my own. I cannot fully explain where this idea came from, but at the time it felt like the right thing to do. So, with Kim's blessing we moved Janet into our home. What I thought Janet needed most was to once again start participating in everyday life. While keeping a structured environment and boundaries was important, I felt it was equally important for Janet to start experiencing some normalcy in her life. And to be honest, she needed to start making new memories and put her old ones in their rightful place. More than anything, Janet needed to start a new chapter in her life, a chapter that empowered her to move forward.

Today, Janet is living a life that is empowered and hopeful. She lives in a small assisted living home where she has built new relationships with her peers. Janet participates willingly in daily activities both inside and outside of her home. Her eyes are bright again and reflect the new light inside of her. Janet's relationship with Kim has been restored and continues to grow in a healthy direction. Janet has also returned to fulfilling one of her most important roles in her family, Grandma. She proudly wears a necklace around her neck that says so. I recently had an opportunity to share with Janet how grateful I am that she and Kim are part of my life. She returned those same feelings to me, then wrinkled up her nose and expressed that she wished we had met on different terms. I told her I would not change anything about our journey because it has led us to this moment together. She smiled, gave me a nod of acknowledgment and we hugged.

Chapter 19

Darkness Before Light

*"When you look into the eyes of your old dog, you
won't see any regret. There is only gratitude for
every moment they have spent with you, hope for
one more adventure, and unconditional love."*
–Yours Truly

S ometimes, a story starts with a very dark chapter but still
ends up having a happy ending. As I write these words it
becomes clear to me just how much I need this reminder. I
wish all stories about people and the animals they love ended this
way. Pearl's happy ending began in a place of deep sadness and
grief. She was not the first member of our pack to suddenly fall
ill. In the nine months before Pearl got sick, our family lost three

dogs. Our beloved Bailey was the first to go. She was my soul dog and if you've been lucky enough to experience this, you understand the magnitude of that loss. But she had lived a good long life. She almost made it to her 14th birthday, which for a Beagle is pretty darn good. Still, she was our son's first dog and because the timing was what it was, she left us shortly after Anthony left the nest. Many times, I had done the math and many times I had morbidly projected this would be the case. However, when it happens, nothing can prepare you for the rawness of that moment.

Because we had not lost a pet up to this point, we had no idea how much it would not only affect us, but the other dogs as well. Sophie was especially impacted by Bailey's death. My husband called her "Nugget" for reasons I can't remember. Maybe it was because she was so small when she came into our lives. She was the only puppy we ever brought home. We knew Bailey needed a friend and thought getting a younger dog would be best. Over the previous 12 years, they had become best of friends, as long as Sophie knew her place, which was always second to Bailey. As Bailey aged, Sophie seemed to understand, and on most days, challenged her a little less to be the pack leader. After Bailey took her last breath, we allowed the other dogs to sniff her, hoping this would help them to understand she was gone. Pearl and Jack didn't seem too interested, but Sophie stayed close until it was time to bury her. She seemed to understand her friend was gone.

Our other two dogs, Pearl and Jack had developed their own special bond over the years. Jack and his "Pearl-friend" were almost always together. After Bailey died, they appeared to be unaffected, but Sophie seemed so lonely without her. I knew we could never replace Bailey, but I thought another friend for Sophie might help us all heal a little. With Sophie being 12, I figured getting an older dog would be a good idea. About a week into my search, I found Winnie, a 7-year-old Beagle and thought she would be the perfect fit. When I spoke with the local rescue she was relinquished to, they told me she had lived a pretty neglectful life. Winnie was extremely overweight due to a thyroid issue because her owner had not sought treatment for her. In that moment, I believed Winnie needed us as much as we needed her. When my husband and I first met her, she was easygoing and mellow, just like Sophie. I brought treats with me just in case she needed a little motivation to get to know us. As soon as she saw them, she tapped her front paws on the ground. Immediately we both became emotional because Bailey had always done this. We referred to this as "tippy-tapping". We took this as a good sign and decided to adopt her. After we brought her home, we lovingly gave her the nickname of "Big Booty Judy" because she was such a chunk. Winnie loved going on walks, playing in the yard and taking naps on the couch. Our pack felt complete again.

As the year was coming to an end, and we reflected on all we had lost but also all that we had gained. We had no clue what was coming next. In a way, I suppose that is what protects us from living in constant fear of the next loss. Sophie was fine on Christmas and enjoyed her special treats just like she always had. And then suddenly, she was not ok. We rushed her to our vet and were given the grim news that she was in full-blown heart failure. It was clear that our vet thought we should euthanize her right then and there. But we just could not wrap our heads around this. We needed more time and we needed Sophie to be given a chance to improve. We were sent home with Lasix and the knowledge that Sophie would probably not get better. My husband Todd was definitely Sophie's favorite person. Just as Bailey was my soul dog, I think Sophie was his. He never stated it in that way, but sometimes words aren't necessary to know these things. He spent that night trying to comfort Sophie. He was up and down with her all night long. In the morning, we both understood that Sophie wasn't going to get better and we needed to put our grief aside and help her. It was New Years' Eve and we were never so happy for a year to come to an end. That night my husband and I bawled and mourned losing our precious Sophie just three short months after losing our beloved Bailey.

As we faced the New Year, in complete disbelief that we had lost our two girls, we remembered who we are. We are the Fabulous Felts Family and we had become experts at turning lemons into lemonade. In fact, when life handed us lots of lemons we sarcastically referred to it as the Felts Factor. It was kind of like Murphy's Law. Over the years, it had become the explanation for why some kind of ridiculous thing had happened to our family. And, believe me when I say, the Felts Factor seemed to be at play big time lately. In this case, it helped us turn disbelief into determination. Knowing we could not possibly handle another death any time soon, we decided to adopt a younger dog. Our intentions were to save another Beagle, but Coco, a ten-month-old Corgi Chihuahua mix stole our hearts instead. We thought her youth was exactly what we all needed. However, what we didn't need were the vet bills for the surgery to correct her botched spay and the cost of the medicine and vet visits for all four dogs when she brought home kennel cough. It took more than a month for everyone to get better. Although Pearl and Jack may never forgive us for that one, we all survived, made a little more lemonade and celebrated that our pack was once again whole.

While Jack and Pearl continued their love affair, Winnie and Coco quickly became the most unlikely of friends. Winnie had lived a solitary life before joining our family and didn't understand all the benefits of being part of a pack. Coco would run circles around Winnie and bark at her, in an attempt to get her to play. Winnie would look at us pitifully not understanding why this crazy little white dog kept doing that. Coco seemed to understand that Big Booty Judy needed to start playing for more reasons than just exercise. Her heart needed it to put those first seven years behind her, be a dog, and have some fun. Coco was determined to teach Winnie the art of a good chase. Once the chase finally began, the joy soon followed. It didn't seem to matter to Winnie that she had no chance of ever catching Coco. She simply enjoyed running with her new friend. Just as Winnie was settling in as part of our family, tragedy struck. Winnie had a lump on her stomach that I had asked our vet about when we first adopted her. She reassured me that it was nothing to be concerned about. Unfortunately, it was large tumor on her spleen that had probably gone undiagnosed for many years. Ironically, the tumor had most likely ruptured during one of her runs with Coco. Within 48 hours of the first sign that something was wrong, we lost her. We saved a 7-year-old Beagle who had never known what it was like to be loved and part of a family. There wouldn't have been enough years left in her life to make up for the first seven that she had survived, but we were going to try. How could the Universe be so cruel to take her away from us just seven months later? This took all of us to a whole new level of broken.

Thankfully, my family does not stay broken for long. When we talked about Winnie, it always came back to wishing we had decided to adopt her sooner and had more time with her. This regret was the catalyst that demanded we not be paralyzed by our grief, but instead take action to save another life. But not just any life, we wanted to find another senior Beagle, so we could honor the memory of Winnie. When my local search found only young dogs, I broadened my search to dogs within 250 miles. When that search also came up empty, I secretly decided to broaden my search to all dogs within 500 miles of Denver. I am aware of how crazy that may sound, but at the time it felt like the right thing to do. That leap of faith found Kiana, a 9-year-old Beagle. Her owner had decided she no longer had time for her, so she relinquished her to the local humane society in Casper, Wyoming. Because of our work schedules, it was impossible for us to make the 300-mile drive during the week. I made it my mission to connect with the director at the humane society, so he would give us the time we needed to make the trip. I poured my heart out to him about our recent losses and how dedicated we were to save a senior dog. He told me how sad it made him when people dropped off senior dogs and that it was happening more often. Together, we had the opportunity to give Kiana a better ending, and so we did. Ten days later we made the four-hour drive and met her. She was so full of life, and just like Winnie, she tippy-tapped when she saw the treats. Again, we took this as a good sign and adopted her. As a way to leave her old life behind and to honor the old girls before her, we combined the names of Sophie, Bailey and Winnie and renamed her Sadie. When she heard it for the first time, she tilted her head to the side, wagged her tail and seemed to understand all the love that came with her new name.

As our pack once again felt complete, I could not shake this feeling that we had one more hurdle to face. Typically, I am not the kind of person who worries or focuses on doomsday kind of thoughts. But my gut kept telling me I needed to prepare for something big that was about to happen. The more I tried to shake this feeling the stronger it became. I tried to convince myself that what I was experiencing was grief and the fear of more loss. For a short time, I allowed myself to be comforted by this explanation. My intuition has always been strong and as a kid I often was confused by how I would think about something happening and then it would actually happen. It would be especially scary for me if those thoughts involved someone getting sick or dying. As an adult, I began to realize that this was a kind of gift and could be used to help me connect with people. It seemed like the more I was open to these thoughts the more they became clear to me. In nursing, I often used my intuition as an additional tool to help me understand what was really going on with my patient. As a nurse, I viewed my intuition as strength, but for some reason, I still struggled with this gift on a personal level. Finally, when I could ignore my thoughts no longer and fully allowed my intuition to reveal its message to me, I knew it was about Pearl.

Chapter 20

Saving Pearl

"There was never a night or a problem
that could defeat sunrise or hope."
–Sir Bernard Williams

On the morning we woke up to Pearl panting, I knew this was what had been coming, what I had been trying to ignore for so long. As we drove to the vet, my mind was filled with thoughts of Winnie. After several tests, the diagnosis was nearly the same as what Winnie's had been. Pearl most likely had a tumor on her spleen, it was bleeding, and the vet thought it was most likely cancer and the prognosis was grim. Pearl would not survive this, and it would be best to euthanize her to end her suffering. I absolutely could not accept this scenario. Many times after losing Winnie, I had wondered if we should have tried the emergency surgery that our vet said she would not survive instead of euthanizing her. I often replayed that day in my head and felt like we had given up on her future because the vet had told us there wasn't any hope for her. As a nurse it was always my goal to instill hope into my patient's lives no matter what the diagnosis is. This was the second time our vet was completely shutting off any chance of hope. She had no definite clinical data that told her this was cancer, yet she was ready to give up. Then it hit me. If this scenario involved my son or my husband, I would never accept this diagnosis and outcome. I would keep fighting for them and do whatever I could to save them. And I surely would get a second opinion.

To get that second opinion, I needed to buy Pearl some time. The second unlikely diagnosis our vet gave us was an infection in Pearl's gut. So why not treat that? I told her that we were not ready to euthanize Pearl, needed antibiotics, and wanted to get more tests done to verify the cancer diagnosis. She looked a bit stunned and reluctantly agreed to give us the antibiotics but told us they probably would not work. What she didn't realize was that I was done with her and her "can't do" attitude. Pearl deserved a doctor that would fight for her. I saw this as an opportunity for me to use my experience as a nurse to help Pearl. As nurses, we don't need to have all the answers; we just need to know where to find them. We also know that when dealing with any illness, especially cancer, your medical team can dramatically impact a positive outcome. It was true that at this moment I definitely did not have answers and quite frankly was a bit intimidated by the whole veterinary arena. If Pearl was going to have a chance at beating this, I needed to find someone that could help me with a crash course in canine medicine and unafraid to think outside of the box. Luckily, I had met that person just a few short months before.

When I first met Tammy, I knew she was my husband's second cousin by marriage, a veterinarian, and that she had not been feeling well for quite some time. She was in Denver to seek medical treatment at National Jewish. Tammy lived in Florida and I felt if she was coming all this way to see specialists, her condition must be quite serious. My only knowledge of her illness was that her lungs had been compromised by many infections and the source of these infections was still a mystery. She was here with Karen, Todd's cousin whom I absolutely adored. Karen had married Tammy's dad James and when he suddenly passed away years later, Karen and Tammy had become closer. When we met them for dinner, I could see the concern in Karen's eyes as Tammy told us about all she had been through. National Jewish had put her through various tests and at the end of the day there seemed to be more knowledge about her condition, but no definite diagnosis or treatment plan. As we parted ways that day, I prayed that she would beat whatever was causing her to be so very sick. Because I knew she was not well, I hesitated to reach out to her, but my need to help Pearl compelled me to.

During our first conversation, Tammy immediately agreed with my decision to get a second opinion. After sharing Pearl's onset of symptoms, current condition and lab results, Tammy told me she didn't think Pearl had cancer. But, to figure out exactly what was going on, we would need to move forward with more diagnostics. Currently, Pearl was not eating or drinking and appeared to be miserable. Part of me felt guilty, like I was only prolonging her suffering. This feeling was holding me back from being totally committed to moving forward. Tammy gave me the opportunity to talk about these feelings and helped me turn my apprehension into action. For the first time since Pearl became sick, I was feeling hopeful and much more confident about using my nursing skills to help her. Turns out human and canine medicine have a lot more crossovers than I realized. Dehydration is one of them and was the first thing we needed to tackle. With Tammy's instructions I began giving Pearl subcutaneous fluids in the back of her neck. Each bolus was 250cc and she looked like the Hunchback of Notre Dame afterwards. She tolerated this much better than any human would have and started to perk up. Shortly after each treatment, she would to eat small amounts of chicken and rice. Clearly, Pearl was not ready to quit, and clearly, I needed to find another vet.

With Tammy's guidance, I searched for another practice that could help us with a definitive diagnosis for Pearl. During my very first phone conversation with Cherished Companions I spoke with Chelsi. She conveyed an exceptional amount of empathy for Pearl. It was as though she had been her patient for many years, not a dog she didn't know. This vet's approach to finding a diagnosis was also completely different than the previous vet. They believed that testing should be affordable, so more money can go towards treatment and more animals can be saved. What a remarkable concept! I scheduled Pearl for an abdominal ultrasound but was told it couldn't be done for a few days because only Dr. Melanie performed this test. Although I was a bit disappointed about the delay, I also understood that having an expert do the test was our best shot at accurate results. Plus, Dr. Melanie would meet with me immediately following the test to go over those results and formulate a plan of action for Pearl.

When I arrived at Cherished Companions, my anxiety level was at an all-time high. As I walked in, I was greeted warmly, just as they had done on the phone. Chelsi, the vet tech who had patiently listened to my saga about Pearl, immediately introduced herself. This practice obviously understood the value of customer service and how important first impressions are. Chelsi exuded the perfect blend of kindness and confidence. The more we went over what would happen that day, the more I felt my anxiety disappear. She had paid close attention to every detail I told her on the phone about Pearl. She understood Pearl's history and that because she came from a puppy mill type of environment being confined stressed her out big time. She promised me that it was absolutely no trouble to keep Pearl in the back without being confined and they would do whatever was necessary to limit any additional stressors for her. I expressed my gratitude for their willingness to go the extra mile for Pearl and as I left I knew this was the right place to seek a diagnosis for her.

After what seemed like days verses mere hours, I headed back to get the news. Once again, I felt reassured as the staff immediately told me that Pearl was fine and had tolerated the procedure without any issues. It became apparent to me that they viewed the animals they cared for as their patients, but the people who bring them as their customers. With this mindset, they anticipated the needs of the animals but also were proactive to meet the needs of the people. They seemed to understand that establishing a relationship with both patients and customers was vital to the success of their practice. As Dr. Melanie walked into the exam room it became obvious that she was the champion of this practice. Her kindness radiated through her eyes and smile as she introduced herself. She confirmed the ultrasound did show a mass on Pearl's spleen, and she also gave me the good news that the rest of her abdomen looked normal. She was very optimistic that performing a splenectomy would most likely cure Pearl. She hoped that the mass on the spleen was just a hematoma and not cancer. Although she would not know until it was removed and biopsied, she felt pretty confident it most likely was not cancer. For every question and concern I had, she gave me answers that were realistic but also hopeful. I asked Dr. Melanie "If Pearl were your dog what would you do?" Her answer was immediate, she would perform the splenectomy. She quickly added that she wanted to help Pearl but also understood that this was my decision. I left that exam room feeling educated and empowered to help Pearl. I could not have asked for anything more from Dr. Melanie. She was truly the answer to my prayers.

Over the next few days, we finalized all the arrangements in order for Pearl to have the splenectomy. There were many options we needed to consider regarding the care both during and after her surgery. First, was the possibility that Pearl may need a transfusion. Tammy suggested we ask if one of our other dogs could be a donor, as it would help cut costs. Dr. Melanie agreed to this and we nominated Jack as the best candidate for this roll. His blood type didn't have to match hers because in canine medicine there is normally no reaction with the first transfusion a dog has. We thought Jack was the best choice because he and Pearl had such a close bond. As her donor, he would be by her side and we thought this might bring some comfort to her. We also agreed that I would do her post-op recovery at home rather than have her stay overnight at the office. One of the final decisions I had to make was signing the DNR in case Pearl coded during surgery. Strangely this one was easy because I refused to believe that we had gone through all of this only to have Pearl's final chapter end with her dying during surgery.

On the day of surgery, I could not have been more confident that Dr. Melanie and her team would prevail. I believed each of them had a connection with Pearl and would go to any lengths to help her. I also knew that there were a lot of people praying for Pearl, Dr. Melanie and her team that day. My gratitude for all the support for Pearl filled my heart completely, leaving no room for any fear. The fear of losing Pearl was gone because I finally realized that the fear I had been feeling was being afraid to take action. And now, for the first time in many weeks, there was nothing more I needed to do. When Dr. Melanie called to tell me that the surgery was over and Pearl was ok, my heart soared. Everything had gone exactly as planned with no complications. She anticipated we would have biopsy results in a few days confirming Pearl did not have cancer. Pearl and I woke up early on post op day one to the most beautiful sunrise, and I hoped that Pearl would be able to enjoy many more sunrises. My heart was filled with gratitude once more for all the people who had not given up on this little dog. The biopsy came back negative, just as Tammy and Dr. Mel had thought it would. Pearl has seen more than 365 sunrises since that day. Her happy ending includes ice cream twice a year; once on her birthday and another on her cure day.

Chapter 21

More Than Enough

*"Three grand essentials to happiness in this life are something
to do, something to love, and something to hope for."*
–Joseph Addison

F or nearly twenty years I allowed myself to believe I didn't
have enough ability to retain information to be able
to successfully complete nursing school. Before that, I
believed I wasn't a good enough wife. As a child, there came a point
when I also began to believe I wasn't a good enough daughter. In
all of these scenarios I allowed fear and self-doubt to control me.
I realize now that I was always more than enough but convinced
myself I wasn't. My self-limiting thoughts and fear held me back
from so much. Over the years I have heard many patients, nurses,

CNAs, and other medical professionals minimize their worth. I hope this chapter will enlighten and empower anyone who has ever thought they were not enough.

No matter where you are on your journey, you are more than enough, right now. Whether you are a care-seeker or care-giver, you are deserving of all the universe has to offer. Everything you need to succeed is already within you. The moment you were born your life was full of promise, hopes and dreams. If something happened that took that away from you, it is time to get it back. Maybe someone told you that you weren't good enough or would never amount to anything. Maybe you decided this for yourself. No matter what caused you to come to this conclusion, it is time for you to recapture who you truly are.

Understanding who you are and knowing your true path is the first step to realizing your full potential. So many times we get locked into being what we think we should be rather than simply allowing ourselves to fully be who we really are. Self-limiting thoughts and fear definitely contribute to this. Allowing other people to define our worth doesn't help either. Most of us are guilty of this from time to time. However, some of us, including myself, have let this stop us from experiencing all life has to offer.

I cannot tell you how many times I have heard the words "I'm just a nurse" or "I'm just a CNA." Subconsciously I think there is an underlying element of fear of not being enough in this statement. Every time this is spoken it minimizes that person's value. This way of thinking also affects our patients. When we minimize our value it takes away our power to be advocates. This further perpetuates the feeling of being powerless for the patient. They're looking to us for support and advocacy and we basically tell them we have no power to do so. It's time for us, as healers to step up and fully understand the importance of our worth.

For me, stepping up into my power began with facing fear and taking action. I found that taking even the smallest step would help cancel out fear. With each step I created more momentum and felt less afraid and more motivated to take another step. Before I knew it, I was taking bigger steps and facing more fear. During moments of hesitation, I began to realize I had a choice to face fear and take action or let fear paralyze me. Honestly, I was sick and tired of letting fear have control over me so I made it my motto to Face Fear and Take Action.

In any part of your life where you feel a bit fearful, it is likely some change may be needed. When thinking about change and moving forward I like to think of it this way. There are just two choices. Either find a solution or find acceptance. Sometimes acceptance can actually be the solution. I think it also helps you decide whether or not something really needs to be changed. Is the fear you're feeling because you need to grow or is it because you need to accept where you are? This can be the tricky part. Sometimes we push when we actually need to pause.

If you have the overachiever gene, you're probably likely to be more comfortable pushing than pausing. This is true for me and it took me quite awhile to realize that as long as I was pushing I could be fearless. However, during moments of pause the fear began creeping into my thoughts. The truth is that the fear is always there but as long as I stay busy I keep it at bay. If that sounds at all remotely familiar to you, get ready to have your mind blown when I share a little secret with you. Our fear will continue to chase us until we have the ability to pause and become best friends with it.

I realize that becoming best friends with your fear may sound a little strange and scary at first. But if you start to see fear as a friend instead of a foe it completely changes your relationship with it. A foe is always out to get you and keep you from winning. A friend, especially a best friend, can motivate you and challenge you to become more than you ever thought possible. Imagine what your life would be like if fear could be that kind of friend. Instead of fear paralyzing you it could fuel you and guide you to be everything you have always wanted to be.

In order for fear to become fuel you've got to face it and embrace it as part of your life. This doesn't mean you accept living your life in a constant state of fear. It means just the opposite. Use fear as a tool to guide you and help you grow. Or use the fear of not being enough to help you pause and take note of all you actually are. Whether you need to push or pause fear can be used as a compass to show you where to direct your attention. Rather than avoid something that elicits fear, try seeking out these things and explore them.

Anytime we explore something that makes us feel uncomfortable we tap into our future potential. If we move through the fear and being uncomfortable we can access all the possibilities that are on the other side. This is where we can clearly see that all we need is already inside of us. We are already more than enough we just haven't realized it yet. Once we experience this new reality we get to enjoy how awesome it feels to be living an authentic life. One that is full of hope and has endless possibilities.

This is where your true life's purpose awaits you. It is a place where your wildest desires can be fulfilled. Where unconditional love and endless amounts of hope reside. Doesn't that sound amazing? And think about this. All of that is already inside of you just waiting to be experienced. So what are you waiting for? How many more days, weeks or years will you let pass by before you realize you are enough? It's time to face your fear, embrace it as your new friend, and get on with living the awesome authentic you!

Chapter 22

Mystery Diagnosis

"The human body experiences a powerful gravitational
pull in the direction of hope. That is why the patient's
hopes are the physician's secret weapon. They are the
hidden ingredients in any prescription."
–Norman Cousins

T his chapter is dedicated to anyone who has ever had a medical problem and didn't receive the care they rightfully deserved. There are numerous reasons why this is happening in healthcare. I think it has always been an issue. Medicine can still be very black and white. We count on clinical data to make a diagnosis to treat the patient effectively. That's a wonderful thing unless the clinical data shows negative test results. This seems to be when the negativity and doubt about the patient begins.

When my son was in preschool, long before I was a nurse, he came down with fifth disease. This is also known as "slapped cheek" rash due to the redness of the child's cheeks. Being exposed to the parvovirus B19 causes it. It is considered a common skin rash in children and not a big deal. My son had all the typical symptoms of low-grade fever, red cheeks, a bit of a headache and a rash. Many kids in his class also came down with this virus. Our doctor told us not to worry and he would be back to himself in seven to ten days. Anthony seemed unaffected by the virus and actually thought he looked cool because his cheeks looked like his favorite Pokémon Pikachu.

Just as our doctor told us, Anthony was back to school in no time without complications. Our life carried on and we got back to our regular busy schedule. About a week later I began to feel really run down. I attributed it to burning the candle at both ends. I thought I just needed to take better care of myself and vowed to try to get a little more sleep. Within days though I knew I was getting really sick. At first it felt like a cold, but quickly became very intense with body aches. Then the unbearable joint pain began. I figured I must have the flu.

When the joint pain didn't go away I went to my doctor. He ran a CBC and the results were unremarkable. He concluded I must have a virus and perhaps it was indeed the flu. He told me I needed rest and hydration. I asked if I could have something to help with the joint pain because Tylenol and Advil were not doing much. I will never forget the look on my doctor's face. He seemed puzzled trying to decide if he should give me a narcotic.

His answer was to come back in two weeks if I wasn't better. I went home without any means of relief from the joint pain. I felt so incredibly defeated.

When two more weeks passed, and I literally had to crawl up my steps to get to my bedroom because I could no longer walk up my stairs I was really scared. I called my doctor and made another appointment. This time he tested me for Lupus and Rheumatoid Arthritis. When those tests also came back negative, my doctor seemed even more skeptical. Again, I explained how much pain I was in and again I left my doctor's office without any diagnosis or treatment. I was beginning to feel pretty hopeless.

When I thought the pain would make me lose my mind, I knew I had to get a second opinion. After seeing a second doctor who basically performed the same tests again producing negative results, my mental health was questioned. This doctor actually had the nerve to say what the first doctor was thinking. Basically, I was a hypochondriac, because with all negative test results there was just no medical explanation for the type of pain I claimed I had. Now I was angry. How dare he make this type of accusation about me. I was a woman who prior to this situation had been perfectly healthy. I literally only saw my doctor for my yearly exam.

Now even more desperate, I turned to my friend Joyce for help. She encouraged me to make an appointment with her doctor who was a Doctor of Osteopathy and Rheumatologist. During our first appointment he asked me similar questions the other physicians had asked. When he learned the Rheumatoid Arthritis and Lupus tests were negative his line of questions changed. He asked me to tell him about my family. He wanted to know if I had any young children. I told him Anthony was in preschool. The next question he asked me changed everything.

He wanted to know if Anthony or any other child in his class had been diagnosed with fifth disease. This question stunned me. Why would this matter? Fifth disease was a childhood virus. The preschool told us adults couldn't get it. I quickly learned how wrong that information was. Not only could the virus spread to adults, sometimes the effect on adults could be quite severe. The only way to know for certain was to check my titers for the virus. He felt confident in the diagnosis, and for the first time in six months I felt like my doctor believed me. He immediately gave me something stronger for my joint pain and started me on a steroid. I left his office feeling so grateful.

A few days later, he made my diagnosis official. My titers were off the chart for Parvo B19. Even though I was a healthy adult, my body had a hyper reaction to the virus exposure. Finally, I knew the cause of my debilitating joint pain. Although there was no cure for what I was experiencing, my symptoms could have been treated and I would not have suffered for the last six months. I felt so victimized by the previous doctors who saw me and wrote me off as a hypochondriac. It would take another twelve months for all my joint pain to dissipate. For eighteen months my life was made miserable by a virus considered to be nothing more than a common childhood rash.

Although I was miserable for almost two years of my life, I still consider myself to be fortunate compared to other women I know. Joyce also had been diagnosed with Parvo B19 a year before she became my neighbor in Colorado. She too had severe arthritic pain for more than eighteen months. Unlike me though, her pain subsided but never really went away. She has since been diagnosed with Fibromyalgia. A diagnosis that doesn't sit well with her because she believes her pain is still related to Parvo B19 virus she was exposed to nearly twenty years ago. I tend to agree with her.

When my neighbor Elizabeth suddenly became ill eight months ago, I immediately became alarmed when she told me about her symptoms. She described it as feeling like she was getting a cold and then the flu. She told me her joint pain was very intense. Elizabeth has three children. Her oldest son Joey is a teenager and her youngest son Timmy is under the age of five. Her daughter Charlotte is just a baby. Instantly I thought to myself could they have been exposed to the Parvo B19 virus? Joey had recently had flu-like symptoms after going to the doctor's office for a physical. Elizabeth had brought all three kids with her that day. This was a likely place of exposure.

Within five days of the onset of feeling like she was coming down with a cold, Elizabeth also noted both of her younger children having red cheeks. Elizabeth began to decline rapidly. Her fever shot to 103.2, she became tachycardic and was short of breath. She was in and out of the urgent care with no clear diagnosis. During one of those visits she requested to be tested for exposure to the Parvo B19 virus. Her doctor reluctantly agreed to draw the lab because he believed Elizabeth had Rheumatoid Arthritis. I have no doubt his reluctance was simply a matter of being unfamiliar with Parvo B19.

Just ten days after Elizabeth came down with what seemed to be a cold, she was hospitalized with severe right upper abdominal pain. An abdominal CT scan indicated thickened gallbladder walls and she was scheduled for an emergency cholecystectomy.

However, her heart rate was now too low to perform the surgery. As her kidneys began to fail and her belly filled with fluid, the Parvo B19 test results came back. The results were positive. And yet, the medical team continued to look for a more likely cause.

Once Elizabeth's kidneys were stabilized another scan determined she did not need to have surgery. After a full cardiac work up, her doctor concluded she had a heart murmur. Elizabeth had never been told she had a murmur prior to this hospitalization. There was no other explanation given for the tachycardia, bradycardia and severe hypertension she had recently experienced. Although she continued to complain of abdominal pain and the inability to lie flat, the infectious disease doctor told her the Parvo B19 virus had run its course and she just needed to sleep in a recliner. Later that evening she was discharged.

After Elizabeth got home she weighed herself. She was surprised to find out she had gained nearly twenty-five pounds. When she pushed on her belly she could see waves of fluid under her skin. Her blood pressure was also severely high again. She had no choice but to go back to the emergency room. She demanded an abdominal CT scan, which confirmed the ascites that had been present all along. Once again thickened walls of her gallbladder were noted. She was admitted to the ICU and started on Lasix.

Within twenty-four hours, Elizabeth lost twenty pounds of fluid. During this time her cardiologist also told her she had Lyme disease. A diagnosis, which was later, retracted and considered to be an error. My guess is the medical team was still looking for a more likely culprit to blame all of this on. Elizabeth would not have surgery and was discharged with as needed Lasix for the ascites and Procardia for her remaining hypertension. In the end, after two hospitalizations, the only definitive test result was a positive Parvo B19 titer.

You may ask yourself how it is possible for a virus to wreak this kind of havoc on a normally healthy woman. Instead, my question is, how is it possible that her medical team was unable to better serve her during this crisis? For me the answer is disconnection from our patients. As medical professionals, we sometimes allow ourselves to become more connected to the diagnosis we are searching for than the patient. We need to remember the patient was the catalyst, which started our search in the first place. We must begin with human connection and maintain it throughout our course of treatment. To do anything less is to do harm.

Chapter 23

Closing the Gap

"As long as we have hope, we have direction,
the energy to move, and the map to move by."
–Chinese Proverb

s I write these words, our world seems to be full of gaps. These gaps have caused many people to separate and divide. There are gaps in equality, gender, race, and age. The list goes on. Each gap creates a group of people who potentially fall victim to the gap and others who potentially promote the gap. It seems that there is always an agenda these days. I find myself being cautious about the words I choose to use so I do not run the risk of offending anyone. However, I can no longer remain silent about this epidemic.

At this point, you as a reader are probably pretty aware I do not subscribe to being a victim. I have faced many obstacles in my life, both personally and professionally. Although I may have found myself in the victim's seat, I never felt comfortable there. I honestly don't think any human being does. No matter what it may look like, no matter what an individual may seem to gain by being a victim, deep down inside I believe all human beings would never intentionally chose this position. This may be something we have to agree to disagree on.

One of the main reasons I wanted to write this chapter is because of my son. He is twenty-three, a senior in college and a Millennial, oh my. Despite all he may be facing, I absolutely believe his future is bright. Some of you may think I'm delusional. If so, let's agree to disagree again for just a moment. I believe his future is bright because I believe in Anthony and his ability to survive and thrive. He didn't have a perfect childhood, he was not raised in a wealthy household and he often faced challenges at school. What he did have were parents who put him first, supported him and always loved him unconditionally.

Imagine if all children grew up knowing unconditional love. Imagine if all parents who had not grown up with it still had the ability to break the cycle and give this gift to their children. The healing to follow would leave a huge impact on our future. The kind of impact that could fill in the gaps we face today. Children could grow up knowing the color of their skin, gender and sexual orientation does not define them or keep them from achieving anything they dreamed of. These things, the things no child has control over would no longer control their future. For this future to be realized, we must start finding ways to close the gap, right now, today.

Whether you are a parent currently raising your children, or someone who never intends to have children, you matter. You may be a nurse, doctor, certified nurse assistant, or you may not be in the medical field at all, you matter. Maybe you've been victimized in some way, or maybe you have had a perfect life, you matter. Each of us matters and I believe we need to focus on closing the gaps that divide us. Judgmental comments, eye rolling, and finger pointing only fuels hatred and strengthens the gap. Our world is not made up of them or us. We are all in this together, like it or not.

If you happened to roll your eyes during that last paragraph, I forgive you. At this point, we may still have to agree to disagree. I'm hopeful at the end of this chapter we may be a little closer to agreeing on more than we disagree on. That is where this all starts. You must make an agreement with yourself about your future. Do you want it to be a future full of human connection or would you rather live a dysfunctional, disconnected life? The choice is yours, no matter what has happened to you. If you're currently in the victim's seat, there is always a way out. The good news is, you don't have to figure this out on your own.

Each one of us has the power to help each other and ourselves. Each of us has strengths and challenges. We may seem different to one another, but we have more in common than we give ourselves credit for. Too many times we allow our differences to shine more brightly than our commonalities. When this happens, we do not see a true reflection of the human being in front of us. These differences often show up in ugly thoughts, language and labels.

Whether we think them or say them, the damage is done. A choice has been made. We chose judgment over unconditional love.

Most of us grew up being taught to follow the golden rule: Treat others the way you want to be treated. It wasn't about who or what was right or wrong. It was a guideline used to stay in harmony with those around us. Such a simple concept, yet it seems anything but simple these days. The disharmony only widens the gap. When the gap widens we become further disconnected from our humanity. Dehumanization in healthcare is just one symptom of this worldwide epidemic. Those of us who are in healthcare have an extraordinary opportunity to heal our world, one patient at a time.

We must first acknowledge who we are and why we made the leap to this profession. Maybe you're like me and dreamed of being in healthcare all your life. Maybe you fell into the role you're in now. Maybe somewhere along the line you lost your "why". Now is the time to remember. Each of us will have our why and those whys may be very different from someone else's. This is not a time to judge our peers for their why. This is where the unconditional love and human connection begins. If we can't accept each other, how in the world will we accept our patients?

Let's begin by seeing a true reflection of our peers. See the person, not their degree. The letters behind someone's name is not an indication of his or her value. We are all human beings with different levels of education and experience. For some of us, connecting with someone else might be our strength. For others, we have to try a bit harder. The reality is, we all have the ability to connect. So, if the ability is there in us all, it comes down to choice. Personally, I cannot imagine choosing not to connect with another human being. If by chance you are this type of person, I strongly suggest finding a different profession. If you just rolled your eyes, again I forgive you, but this is further indication you may need to find a new job.

Think about someone who means the world to you. Someone you love unconditionally. This is how we should be approaching our peers and patients. Maybe easier said than done, at least initially. But with practice, this can become a more natural approach. For me, my son and my husband are the people I think of. So, when I meet a new peer or patient I remind myself that he or she is someone's child. This instantly opens my heart to this person. I may see a child who has been loved unconditionally or I may see a child who seeks this type of love. Either way, I am seeing a human being who is seeking care or a human being who wants to give care.

With women, I often find instant rapport when I connect with them as a daughter, sister or wife. It's true that misery loves company, but it is also true there is power in comradery. When the person we are caring for or seeking care from see us as someone they can instantly identify with, it begins a meaningful connection. Once this connection is established, we can move on as a team and face whatever it is together. Safety in numbers is real and sometimes all someone needs to move forward is to know they are not alone.

Now that you have a connection with the person you're caring for or seeking care from, you should begin to feel a little harmony. Which in my experience makes the next step in closing the gap a little less intense. No matter how many ideas we have about what care should look like, it is also important to give the other person the opportunity to share their ideas. As a giver of care, I think it's vital we remember whose life will be most impacted by the care. If I am receiving the care I must advocate for the care I expect to receive. This exchange must be done in a mutually respectful way and yes, sometimes there may be a need to agree to disagree to move forward.

In the forward movement, or the mutual participation of the team is where the momentum grows. Any time care-givers and care-seekers work together to improve a patient's health, humanity is restored to healthcare overall. Our care plan becomes more about the human involved and less about their history or physical diagnosis. Of course, this clinical information is necessary for many reasons. I'm simply stating that it shouldn't be the most important thing we consider when giving or receiving care. If we are truly giving or receiving care based on the whole person there is so much more to consider.

When we work with one another as peers, care-givers and care-seekers, it leads us to empowered care. Being empowered further liberates us all from the negative thoughts and ideas which leads us to gap mentality. Instead of being fearful and feeling out of control, we are exactly the opposite. When we take control of care, without fear of judgment, the gap begins to disappear. This is where true continuity of care can begin.

Next time you see a care-giver or care-seeker who looks like a 23-year-old Millennial college kid, please stop yourself from judging too quickly. That human in front of you is someone else's child. Whether this person had the good fortune to experience unconditional love or is still waiting for it, they need you. My grandma Dorothy always taught me that it is better to give than to receive. She was one of the most generous people I will ever know. She also died prematurely because she didn't receive the medical care she was so deserving of. Let us all as care-givers and care-seekers both give and receive the unconditional love and care each of us deserves.

Chapter 24

Opportunity For All

"My friends, love is better than anger. Hope is better than fear. Optimism is better than despair. So, let us be loving, hopeful and optimistic. And we'll change the world."
–Jack Layton

My hope for you, whether you are a care-giver or care-seeker, is that this book has touched your heart in some way. My intention for sharing the events of my life is to connect with you, one human being to another. We all have life experiences that have the ability to connect or disconnect us. We all have different points of view, which have the power to do the same. I ask you to choose. Choose to put aside thoughts that may disconnect you from another human being. Choose the power of Human Connection.

For all the care-seekers reading this book, I want you to know that I understand sometimes your diagnosis seems to precede you. I realize this perception isn't fair and that is what I want to change more than anything. In order for this to happen, I need your help. I need you to show the care-givers involved in your care that there is an amazing human standing behind the diagnosis they're so focused on. I need you to find ways to connect with them and engage them, so they really see you. I know this isn't always easy, especially when you don't feel well. But I need you to try. I promise if you keep trying, they will see you.

Sometimes as care-seekers we give up. I understand that too because I've been there. I've given up. Now, I understand that acceptance of a situation is okay, but giving up isn't. No matter what health issue you are facing, please don't give up. Because when you give up, you become disconnected and it becomes that much harder for a care-giver to see you. Sometimes, when you're disconnected it seems like you don't care. And when a care-giver who has very little left to give sees that you don't care it's easier for them not to care. This may sound harsh, but if we are being honest, it happens.

So, don't allow your diagnosis to disconnect you. Remember who you were before that moment, before the diagnosis cast a shadow over you. You were strong. You did "fill in the blank". You were proud of "fill in the blank". You used to always talk about "fill in the blank". Guess what? You are still a wonderful human being and all that comes with you is still there. You just have to choose. Choose to remember yourself and let all of that glorious

YOU connect with the caregiver before you. And if at first they don't see you, just be patient, they soon will.

For those of us who are on the care-giving end of this relationship, we must accept our responsibility and find ways to connect with the people who are seeking care from us. Let's face it, we chose to be in this position. They did not. We get paid to be here and they are the ones paying. Without the care-seeker there is no need for the care-giver. Remember that next time you enter a room and meet the human attached to the diagnosis that preceded them on the chart you're looking at. While a diagnosis helps us understand what's going on, there is nothing more important than the human being in front of you.

Just for a moment allow yourself to really be present with your patient. Then ask yourself "What do I see?" What is it you notice about this person that may help you establish a connection? Ask yourself "What is their blank?" They used to do "fill in the blank"? They were so proud of "fill in the blank". Maybe their blank is sitting in the room with them. What was this person's life like before this moment with you? I'm pretty sure they were not sick and broken like their current diagnosis may indicate. They had a life, one that you can help them get back to more quickly if you connect with them. I promise if you try to see them, they will show you who they really are.

When a care-giver seeks to positively impact the life of the person they are caring for, they must start with Human Connection. When you connect on a human level you are more invested in your patient's outcome. People can feel this, and they are much more likely to be honest and open with you. This leads to improved cooperation and compliance. Care-givers who have the ability to connect with their patients also tend to experience less burn out. Once true Human Connection is established, hope begins.

Once hope has sparked, care-seekers have the Opportunity not only to be seen, but also to be heard. Now is the time to use your voice. I understand this may feel a little awkward at first. Most care-seekers aren't given the time to talk about how they are feeling emotionally. Consideration isn't always given for the toll their illness has taken on them. This must change, and care-seekers must be brave enough to use this Opportunity to impact their care. This is when you tell your care-givers what is important to you and what you want for your future. You must take the lead on this one.

Taking the Opportunity to lead your care-giver changes the equation completely. Instead of the status quo, which is basically the care-giver telling the patient what is going to happen next, the care-seeker can be in the driver's seat. This is your moment to shine. Remember your "fill in the blank" and use it to fuel your determination to change the way your care-giver sees you. Step out in front of your diagnosis and give your care-giver the chance to see you and listen to what matters most to you.

For care-givers, taking this step forward in hope may be a little tough for you. We are so accustomed to taking the lead with care-seekers. It starts when we get report, which is always care-giver to care-giver. Before we ever lay eyes on the person we will be caring for, we already have a picture of them in our minds. Sometimes this picture is accurate and sometimes it is not. The care plan may have already been initiated based on diagnosis only. This needs to change. If you are open to really listening to your patient and giving them the Opportunity to tell you what is important to them, it can change.

With our Human Connection established and fully utilizing the Opportunity to communicate with one another, it's time for action. Human Connection and Opportunity are necessary in developing hope, but they alone cannot move it forward. Action with Participation is what propels hope. I like to think this part of hope is our action agreement. Care-givers and care-seekers can find meaningful unity during this step. When we are aligned in our goals of care, and participating together to reach those goals, this is where the healing really begins.

Healing is the final step in achieving and sustaining hope. The healing I am referring to is Empowerment. When care-givers and care-seekers are empowered it's a total game changer. Obstacles that put a halt on care are no longer a challenge. Empowerment completely negates fear and when fear is taken out of medicine, miraculous outcomes are possible. It is time to restore humanity in healthcare. It is time for a prognosis of hope.

The story can't end here though, because to end it here means we go no further. This needs to be the beginning. I want to start a revolution that truly leads to H+O+P=E. Care-givers and care-seekers must understand they both need to take action in order for this idea to move forward. It's one thing to read a book and align with the message. But that is not going to restore humanity to healthcare. We need to take steps to ensure this message creates true change in the way medicine is delivered. The first way to take action is to simply start a dialogue with another person. This person may be a colleague, peer, friend or complete stranger. Starting a conversation and sharing ideas about this concept is key.

Once more people become familiar with the idea that we can take control of our healthcare system, I believe things will really begin to change. I plan on doing my part to share these ideas with key people in the healthcare system. I want home care agencies, assisted livings, hospitals, rehabs, hospice and home health agencies to use this model to deliver care. Every person who seeks care should begin to expect and demand this model of care. When care-seekers speak up, the care providers will listen. When care-givers also speak up and request this new model of care to be used, this is when the culture of medicine will change.

We also need things to change in our communities. Instead of offering families and care-givers support groups, let's offer Empowerment groups. Please don't get me wrong. I am not in any way trying to disrespect support groups. However, when folks leave after an hour or so of being supported, I fear that many of them fall back into the same hopeless place they were in. Maybe if we promoted the H+O+P=E model people would be able to actually move forward from their place of despair. Instead of support that acknowledges their problems, we give them a plan of action.

The way we educate our care-givers also needs to change BIG time! Nurses, doctors and CNAs are primarily taught about the clinical side of medicine. Yes, there have been some strides made focusing on dignity, respect and bedside manner. But that only addresses the dehumanization in healthcare on the surface. The deeper root cause of this epidemic is human disconnection. Until we can BEGIN with Human Connection, and choose to put the diagnosis second, healthcare will continue with the same status quo.

Complacent individuals allowed our healthcare system to get to this point. That may be tough to hear, but I believe it is a true statement. The good news is that Empowered care-givers and care-seekers have the ability to end this. I cannot do this alone, nor do I want to. I am asking for you, whether you are a care-giver or care-seeker to stand with me and be part of the Prognosis H+O+P+E Revolution. We CAN and we WILL restore humanity to healthcare.

Want to Join the Revolution?

Email: PrognosisHopeRevolution@gmail.com
Website: PrognosisHopeRevolution.com

In Memory of

Shelley Moriston

As I write these words on the one-year anniversary of your angel day, I still find myself in disbelief. How could a flame as bright as yours be extinguished so tragically? Through my tears I can still see your bright smile and crystal blue eyes. Those eyes saw something in me when I was unable to. You fully believed in my message of hope when I was just beginning to.

To know you was to love you. You were so many things to so many people. But perhaps your greatest gift to this world was your ability to teach and inspire your students. During one of our many heartfelt conversations, you told me that you believed nurses could make the biggest impact through teaching. I believe it was your life's mission to teach and change the world through your students.

Although your time here on earth was much too short, your impact spreads far and wide. I have no doubt that every student you encouraged has positively impacted the world in some way or another. You taught us all that one person can make a difference in the lives of so many. I am forever grateful for the impact you made on my life. Because of you Shelley, I am brave enough to tell my story and share Prognosis H+O+P=E with the world.

About the Author

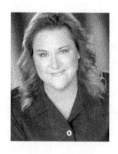

Angie Felts is passionate about human connection and restoring humanity to healthcare. As founder of PrognosisHopeRevolution.com—the premier site focusing on care-giver and care-seeker collaboration and empowerment—she speaks and writes regularly on this powerful topic.

As a registered nurse with experience in med/surg, mental health, long term care, hospice, assisted living and home care, Angie understands the challenges nurses face today. It is her personal goal to empower 1,000,000 nurses through the Prognosis Hope message.

She is also a business owner with more than twenty-five years of sales and marketing experience. Her focus is on community collaboration and developing meaningful partnerships that have a lasting positive impact on the people she serves.

While her work is very rewarding and important to her, it is her son, Anthony and husband, Todd that mean the most. As a CNA, life partner and business partner, Todd shares Angie's passion for human connection and restoring humanity to healthcare.

9 781642 793482